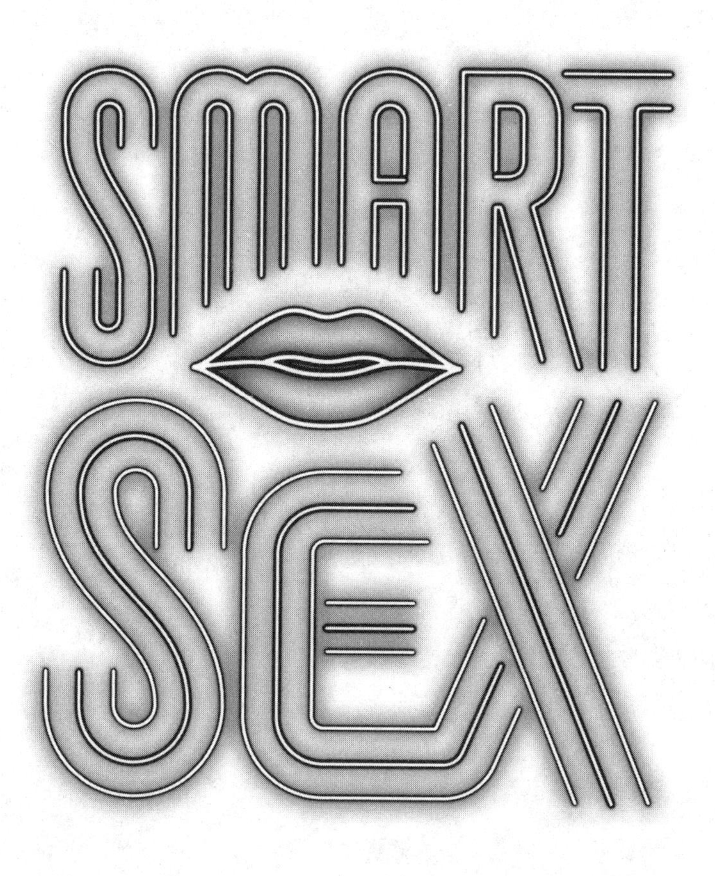
SMART
SEX

DR. EMILY MORSE

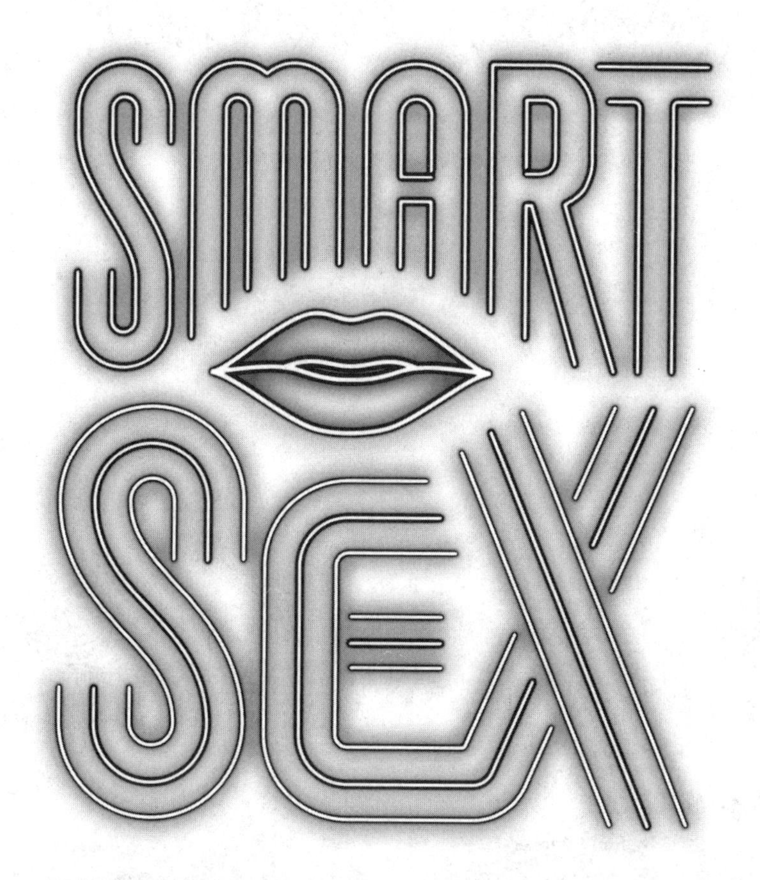

HOW TO BOOST YOUR SEX IQ AND OWN YOUR PLEASURE

ILLUSTRATIONS BY PRISCILLA WITTE

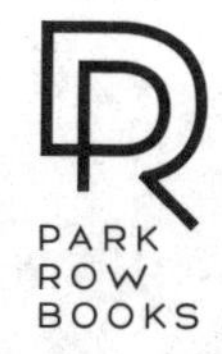

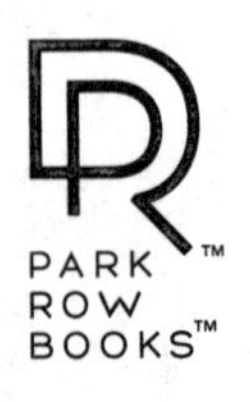

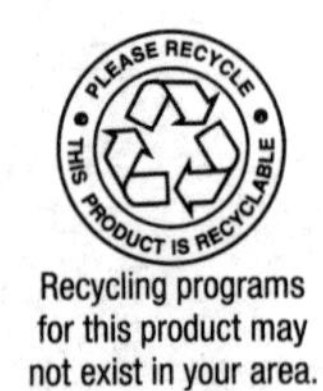

ISBN-13: 978-0-7783-8710-7

Smart Sex

Park Row Books
22 Adelaide St. West, 41st Floor
Toronto, Ontario M5H 4E3, Canada
ParkRowBooks.com
BookClubbish.com

Printed in U.S.A.

I would not be able to write this book without
the support and consistency of my loyal listeners and
the *Sex with Emily* community. This book is a
dedication to your growth, love and Sex IQ.

TABLE OF CONTENTS

INTRODUCTION

Pleasure Is Productive

By the age of thirty-five, many people think that their best sex is behind them, but the exact opposite was true for me.

At that age, I found myself at the end of yet another relationship, feeling beyond frustrated by what felt like a never-ending cycle of dating, entering a relationship, and breaking up. I wondered what the hell was wrong with me and if I was missing a chip or something when it came to sex and relationships.

Of course, by then I'd had good sex. Maybe even great. But every time I met someone, once the thrill of new relationship energy wore off, the sex ceased to be exciting. Back then, I didn't know much about how sex worked and that it was common—and even normal—for attraction to fade once the "honeymoon period" ended. So, when this happened, I figured the relationship had run its course, and before long I was the one who was running.

At that point, I felt in my bones that I could not keep this cycle up forever. But I didn't like either of the two options that I assumed I had to choose between—to accept the fact that hot sex would be a thing of the past only a year or two into a relationship, or to keep starting over with someone new once the sex inevitably cooled.

For the first time, I thought seriously about whether or not there was a third option. Could great sex actually last? And if so, what made it stay hot in the same relationship year after year?

There was also a part of me that wondered what great sex even was, and whether or not I had actually experienced it. Sure, I knew that sex felt good, but when my friends talked about having mind-blowing sex, I just kind of smiled and nodded along. The truth is, I wasn't sure what they were talking about.

What made sex incredible instead of just plain good? Was it having an orgasm every time, having multiple orgasms, or having some sort of miraculous, fierce orgasms? Those things for sure weren't happening for me. My partners pretty much always had an orgasm, but not me. This left me confused, and honestly, a little bit resentful. I assumed that my partners should know how to please me, and I thought it was their fault when they didn't.

Now of course I realize how misguided this was. The truth is that *I* didn't know what I needed to fully enjoy sex. How was anyone else supposed to know? The fact that my partners had no clue that I wasn't orgasming definitely didn't help, either. When I wasn't feeling it, I always faked an orgasm. I put on quite a show, arching my back, moaning, and performing all the moves I'd seen in sexy movies. I cringe looking back now.

So, there I was at thirty-five with little awareness of my own sexuality, no experience communicating with my partners about sex, and the idea that the moderately good-to-great sex I had experienced couldn't last. Quite a recipe for a satisfying sex life, am I right?

I don't blame my younger self, though. The problem that I'm

describing is a cultural one, not an Emily one. Our culture prioritizes denial, self-sacrifice, relentless productivity, and modesty over sexual pleasure. Plus, it presents sex through a defeatist and often shame-riddled lens.

As a result, even my most sex-loving friends seemed to share the tacit understanding that hot sex would be a temporary part of their lives. This often became a self-fulfilling prophecy. I watched people who had once been liberated and experimental with high sex drives devolve into transactional sex lives once they settled into a long-term relationship. I can't tell you how many times I heard, "He has to get his fix, so I force myself to go through with it every two weeks," or, "I always initiated, and they were never into it. I constantly felt rejected, so I just stopped trying."

Spoiler alert—it doesn't have to be this way. I didn't know this for certain yet, but I did have an inkling that I didn't have the full story when it came to sex. How could I, when I talked about it so little, even with my closest friends?

I figured that if I wanted to open up the conversation and learn more about sex, I had to start asking questions.

I sat my most confident and candid friend down and asked her to walk me through an amazing sexual experience—my very first Q and A (of thousands to come) about sex. I asked her the questions I'd always wanted answered: What were her orgasms like? What positions felt the best? What actually happened, moment by moment, that made the sex so mind-blowing?

That conversation led to others. One-on-one impromptu sex chats expanded into group discussions in my apartment in San Francisco. I invited over more friends and interesting strangers with the sole purpose of talking openly about sex and relationships. My goal then—which is still my goal today—was to liberate the conversation about sex.

The discussions were funny and unflinching, and I was learning a ton! I wanted to share this knowledge with more people.

With permission from the participants, I started recording the talks, and eventually I turned them into a podcast.

Podcasts were barely a thing when I launched *Sex with Emily* back in 2005. I had high hopes and low expectations and no idea if anyone would even find the show, but they did—in droves. Right from the beginning, my inbox was flooded with questions about specific acts, fantasies, partner problems, unmet needs, confusion, and loss of desire. I spoke to so many people who were ashamed about sex and had so many questions, but they didn't know where to turn. So, they turned to me—a fellow seeker who was trying to figure this whole sex thing out.

I quickly became obsessed with learning as much as I could about sex and sharing that information with my listeners. It felt incredible when they wrote to me saying that my advice had actually helped improve their sex lives and their relationships. I felt that I had found my calling.

To learn even more, I decided to earn my doctorate in human sexuality—a significant step in reorienting my life around pleasure—and went from asking questions about sex to answering them. Oh, yeah, and I finally started having the best sex of my life.

What I've learned along the way will fill the pages of this book. But my number one takeaway is that we *all* need to reeducate ourselves on sex and pleasure.

Who here remembers their sex ed class in school? I don't know about you, but mine took place in a single hour on a single day in middle school, and instead of learning about communication or consent or, heaven forbid, sexual pleasure, we were mostly taught reasons to fear sex—at least, outside of marriage. I left school that day basically believing that if I had sex, I would probably get a sexually transmitted infection (STI), get pregnant, and maybe even be a bad person. Quite a turn-on!

Of course, so many of us carry that confusion and fear into our adult sex lives and develop shame and embarrassment around sex. This is especially true of single people, who constantly receive the message that the best sex they can hope for is emotionally shallow, pitiful, and disposable—hookups, one-night stands, casual sex, or even a friends-with-benefits situation. I bought into this, too, which is probably why I hopped from relationship to relationship instead of enjoying casual sex, which I now know can be fantastic and fulfilling if we're intentional about it and know what we want from the connection, even if it's temporary.

Yes, it was clear that my issues with sex weren't an Emily problem. But here's the thing—they weren't really a sexual problem, either. Our culture has a problem with pleasure in general. Sexual pleasure is just one kind of pleasure, which includes anything and everything that makes you feel good.

Pleasure is a habit, a practice, and it stimulates our senses: the visual beauty of nature, the sound of a friend's laughter, the scent of a favorite candle, the rich taste of a warm brownie, or the soothing sensations of a massage. This way, it reminds us that we are alive.

Many of us do not even realize how little pleasure we are currently experiencing. We've built our whole lives around avoiding pleasure and starving ourselves of it. We are hustlers, people who "optimize for growth," and get shit done. We have a good day when we complete our checklist and feel self-righteous and productive.

The benefits of pleasure aren't obviously translatable into money, and in our society that makes them worthless. We praise the "superhero" mom who does it all, the people who work the hardest and sacrifice the most, not the ones who take a break midday for a walk in the woods or to indulge in their favorite treat or to give themselves an orgasm. Of course, we feel guilty and selfish when we take time for pleasure (something I *still* struggle with, by the way).

Added to this shame stew is the cultural messaging about the kinds of bodies that deserve pleasure. We're just starting to see this tide shift, but those of us who came of age pretty much at any point before I wrote this book grew up marinated in images about who is worthy of pleasure, which was basically limited to those with white, young, thin, cisgender bodies.

Well, let me just say—screw that. Throughout this book, my goal is to help you unlearn the idea that pursuing pleasure is something that should be limited to certain people or that is inherently selfish, and even that being selfish is bad! I want you to embrace the idea that no matter who you are, you are worthy of experiencing pleasure. End of story.

Not only that, but you owe it to yourself—and to the world—to experience pleasure. It's time to reframe what it means to be productive. By definition, productivity means making intentional choices toward a goal. Well, what if your goal is to be happy, fulfilled, embodied, and joyful? In that case, pursuing pleasure would be the steps you take toward that goal.

By the way, without a life of pleasure and the thrilling, joyful feelings that come with it, you can kiss a life of sexual pleasure goodbye. Once we develop a healthy relationship with pleasure, we know when we're satisfied and when we haven't had enough. That's because pleasure wants to flow freely, without intrusive thoughts of worry, judgment, or fear, and in so doing, it sharpens our intuition around craving and satisfaction—necessary ingredients for sexual pleasure.

Pleasure is abundantly healthy and should have never merged with guilt. If you were once suspicious of pleasure (like I used to be), I hope that by the end of this book, you'll feel confident reclaiming pleasure as your birthright.

That said, don't get it twisted. I'm not calling for all-out hedonism or suggesting that you create a life of pleasure by watching TV for hours on end, eating ice cream for breakfast, lunch, and dinner, and masturbating twenty times a day. I'm obviously exaggerating to make a point, but there is an important distinction between pleasure as presence and pleasure as numbing.

In a moment of fully embodied, mindful pleasure, whether it's when you're having an orgasm or playing your favorite instrument, you are in a state of flow and have no choice but to be present. This is entirely different from disconnecting from our feelings and our bodies by spending hours scrolling on social media, overindulging in alcohol, or spending money we don't have. We're going for the present kind of pleasure. I want you to feel more, not desensitize yourself into feeling nothing at all.

This brings me (finally!) to you. You picked up this book because you want more pleasure, particularly sexual pleasure, and on some level, you know that you deserve it. So, what is holding you back?

Maybe you're afraid that you're "doing" sex wrong, or the sexual spark has died in your relationship and you're desperate to get it back. Maybe you're experiencing physical pain or discomfort during sex, you feel that you orgasm too quickly, or you've never orgasmed at all. Maybe you want to be a better lover and you don't know where to begin. Or maybe you're sexually adventurous and satisfied, but you simply want to learn a few more tricks.

Well, I know one thing for sure. No matter what your question or issue or confusion around sex is, I've got you. Because you already possess the most important quality you need to have a wholly satisfying sex life—you're sexually curious. Whether you're looking to learn how to deliver mind-blowing oral, how to explore a kink, or simply how to talk about sex with a straight face, you're a sexual student. And that open mind and curiosity is all you need to start having the sex of your dreams.

When people like you call or write to me with questions, I only have a few precious minutes to listen and offer advice. I often wish that I could sit them down and chat all day, hear the nuances of their problem, and tackle it on a deep level. Finally, with this book, I have my chance.

This book is for us to spend time together learning all about sex—no-holds-barred. I can give you tips on sexual technique all day long, and you'll find tons of actionable tools in these pages to improve your sex life and develop new skills, but I'm even more excited to go deeper and talk about the psychological layers of pleasure, the blocks that may be holding you back from increasing your pleasure factor, and how to effectively communicate about sex with your partner.

Threaded throughout is my personal philosophy of pleasure so that you can hopefully adjust your thinking around it. What if pleasure wasn't the proverbial devil on our shoulder after all? What if pleasure wasn't tempting us to sin or selfishness, sloth, or greed, or to some general moral failure?

What if it was the angel this whole time?

And how are we going to put that angel to work? To answer that question, buckle up, grab your lube, and open your mind as far as it can go. I'm taking you on a pleasure journey, and here's what you can expect.

First and most important, we're going to learn about Sex IQ—a radical new paradigm that will help you understand yourself as a sexual being and become smarter about sex. The five pillars of Sex IQ are Embodiment, Health, Collaboration, Self-Knowledge, and Self-Acceptance. The more you grow your Sex IQ, the more pleasure you will be able to give and receive.

Next, I'll talk you through the common Pleasure Thieves that can keep us from fully enjoying sex and help you self-diagnose your greediest thieves. To have more and better sex, we first have to identify the forces that are stealing our pleasure and kill them off once and for all.

Whether you're new to it or a seasoned pro, you're going to learn new ways to have solo sex—aka masturbate. Through mindful masturbation, you'll discover new avenues to pleasure that you can use to share with partners and to continue pleasuring yourself.

You'll learn why communication is lubrication. This is one of my most oft repeated pieces of advice for a good reason. It's a critical ingredient for a hot sex life. Vocalizing your desires and requests and feedback about sex—no matter how awkward the topic—can be scary. I get it. These talks can be a relationship killer or they can help bring your sex life to the next level. We'll make sure we're accomplishing the latter.

Yes, you are going to orgasm. The moment you've been waiting for. And whatever orgasms you're currently having—or even if you've never had one—my goal is for you to start having them more frequently and more intensely. I'll explain exactly how orgasm works for both vulva and penis owners, and how you can leverage the arousal process to heighten yours.

You'll take a deep dive (it's so hard not to pun) on oral sex and learn my best techniques to pleasure a penis or a vulva. So many of us struggle to open ourselves up to pleasure in this department, so it's equally important to me to help you become empowered both to give and receive.

After that, we're going to look at how to get radically more pleasure out of some classic sex positions. You may think that you know all there is to know about this, but I promise there are small but seismic changes that will make you reconsider positions you've written off and make old favorites feel new again.

We'll add to our pleasure menu with a sexual act that I get tons of questions about and is laden with taboo: anal sex. I'm talking hygiene, toys, anal orgasms (not a myth), and how to enjoyably explore this mysterious act whether or not you are a beginner.

Next, we'll learn how to explore and play through sex. Pleasure doesn't come in just one flavor—and certainly not just vanilla—so this chapter is a no-judgment-zone exploration of kinks and BDSM (starting with what it even is), power dynamics, and all kinds of play that you may or may not have ever considered.

Finally, we'll discuss alternative relationships, which are becoming more and more popular. Even if this is not for you, it's worth your time to consider all of the options that are available and make an intentional, informed choice.

That's where we're headed. And my hope is that by the time you reach the end of this book, you'll be able to strut into each sexual situation—whether it's a solo session, sex with your partner of twenty years, or a new fling—with a renewed sense of confidence (rather than self-doubt). A sexy kind of tension (rather than anxiety). A sense of discovery (rather than mastery). A sense of curiosity (rather than boredom). And rather than guilt, shame, or any limiting beliefs, an expanded imagination about all the erotic places you can go.

You'll notice that throughout the book I use the terms "vulva owner" and "penis owner" instead of man or woman. This is the language I use across all of my platforms because I want them to be places where everyone feels included. I'm giving advice based on genitals, not gender identity or expression. There is no judgment here. Everyone is welcome.

I've also done my best to be as inclusive as possible and give examples of all different types of relationships. This is really important to me. But the majority of questions that I get do come from heteronormative couples, so you may see slightly more of those experiences reflected in the book.

No matter who you are, my hope is that you'll hit the pleasure reset button and fully own the belief that you deserve pleasure and satisfaction—that you will identify and explore what makes you feel good in your body and start doing more of that.

Even more important, I hope that these pages will help you develop a new mindfulness around sex, so that you can discover how to identify your own unique pleasure and generate more of it. You'll integrate pleasure, including sexual pleasure, into your life regardless of your relationship status. I guarantee that as your sexual self-awareness grows, so will your confidence. You'll finally unlock the pleasure-filled life that you were always destined for. To think that it was right here waiting for you, all this time!

Your eroticism is beckoning. And now, let's answer the call.

1

Boost Your Sex IQ:

The Five Pillars of Your Sexuality

What if I told you that the secret to mind-blowing, earth-shattering sex has nothing to do with your body and everything to do with your mind, that it's to develop a new form of intelligence to become smarter about sex and get to know yourself fully as a unique sexual being? Well, it's true. And that's why I developed a new paradigm to help you understand who you are sexually from a deeper and more holistic perspective—Sex IQ.

Just as the concept of Emotional Intelligence (EQ) helped us understand that attributes such as empathy and emotional regulation account for a unique form of intelligence, Sex IQ teaches us that being a good lover to ourselves and others is its own type of intelligence, too.

Understanding your Sex IQ will impact every area of your life, ushering in a new way of thinking about sex and intimate relationships. By evolving your Sex IQ, you'll be able to easily tune in to what's happening in your own body—and why—and really understand and be intentional about your own sex life. As a result, you will become more confident and able to experience more pleasure.

Your Sex IQ is not a score of how much you know about sex or how good you are in bed. It's not really a score at all. It's a way of comprehending where you are sexually at any given time and tracking how it changes over the course of your lifetime. Along the way, you will become a better lover both to yourself and others.

I developed this paradigm after speaking and working with thousands of people over the years and realizing that most of them come to me looking for a quick fix. They want me to tell them why their sex drive is low, why they can't have an orgasm or maintain an erection, or how to ask their partner(s) to participate in a certain kink or fantasy. They're happy to have gotten the question out of their mouths and want me to recommend a supplement for their libido, a vibrator for orgasms, a pill for erections, or a script to talk to their partner. Then they're ready to move on.

I don't blame these people at all. We're not taught to explore our sexuality, and we see no healthy models of this in our culture. And those quick fixes can work, but they often just act as Band-Aids that temporarily ease the symptoms while masking the root of the problem. For example, you might buy a vibrator that I recommend and start having more orgasms—great!—but still struggle to understand what you need to orgasm in the presence of a partner.

Getting to the root of any issue related to sex almost always requires much more than a quick fix. That's because most of the time a question or issue around sex is about so much more than just sex. The solutions aren't just mechanical—they're usually psychological, emotional, and physical in nature. As a result, two people can ask me the same exact question, but the answer I give each of them will be completely different based on a unique combination of personal factors.

It's the same with almost any type of complex personal issue. Consider anxiety, for example. Everyone experiences some level of anxiety at some point, but the causes and underlying issues vary from person to person. And therefore, the path to overcoming the anxiety will also be different. Whether it's work stress, emotional dysregulation, trauma, or any kind of big life changes, digging deeper to understand the roots of our anxiety is the key to treating it. This is why some may find relief from meditation whereas others need to limit caffeine or end a toxic relationship.

It is very much the same when it comes to sex, but until now, we haven't had a way of talking about or comprehending this. There's no metric for where you are sexually, no clear path to understanding or making sense of what you need to do to fully address any sexual issue that arises.

If you're rolling your eyes right now because you picked up this book to learn a fun new sex position or how to make your partner orgasm, I promise we'll get to all of that. But it's so important to start here first. Even with all of the best sex tips in the world, which of course I have, until you really know who you are when it comes to sex *and why*, you'll never discover your true pleasure potential.

Even more important, googling questions about sex can be extremely limiting or even harmful. When we rely on the inaccurate and incomplete information that's out there, we often come to believe common myths around sex—that our sex life will be over at fifty, that we're inadequate if we have a small penis, or that we're broken if we can only have an orgasm one way or haven't orgasmed at all. Sex IQ clarifies the misinformation and will help clear up these myths and change fixed mindsets around sex.

The goal is not to reach your peak Sex IQ and then check this off your list. You can't ever complete this work. It's a practice to understand where you are sexually in this moment so that you can make necessary changes to continue moving forward, evolving, and enhancing your pleasure.

Growing in each of the Sex IQ pillars does require sustained effort, but it also offers an ongoing reward: a present and future of more pleasure, enhanced intimacy, deeper connections, improved health, and more meaningful relationships, including your relationship with yourself.

Your Sex IQ has nothing to do with whether you're partnered or single or in an unconventional or heterosexual relationship. It also has nothing to do with using your tongue a certain way, mastering a specific position, or knowing how to locate the G-spot. When it comes to smart sex, those things just scratch the surface. To go deeper, we have to become sexually intelligent beings and bring that unique form of intelligence to all of our sexual encounters.

Desire Is a Mental Game

Before we get to the Sex IQ pillars and learn how each of them affects our desire, we need to understand what desire really is.

Most likely, you're reading this book because you want more pleasure in your life, particularly sexual pleasure. No matter where you're starting from, I can almost guarantee that it's not your genitals that are keeping you from the kind of sexual pleasure that you want. It's your brain.

I like to say that our brains are our largest sexual organs. Our brains are where our desire and arousal originate—or don't. Many people don't realize that desire and arousal are two separate things, and they are both key to experiencing sexual pleasure. Desire is simply the emotion of wanting something, while arousal is the physical manifestation of mental or emotional stimulation. When you are physically aroused, your blood pressure, heart rate, breathing, and temperature all go up. If you are a vulva owner, your labia and clitoris fill with blood and become more sensitive. If you are a penis owner, your penis fills with blood, gets harder, and stands up. It's fair to say that desire happens in the mind and arousal happens as a result in the body.

So, sexual pleasure starts with desire, with wanting to have a sexual experience. There's no way around this.

One of the most common questions I get from people is about why they don't feel sexual desire at the drop of a hat like they did when they were younger, or how their partners do, or how they see it happen in movies. In some cases, the lack of immediate desire can lead to guilt for not being ready to go as soon as your partner walks in the door. It can also lead to insecurities or frustrations by the partner experiencing more rapid desire. Ultimately it can become difficult to navigate and partners can withdraw from the encounter.

We owe a lot of this confusion to the fact that we only recently began learning about the nature of desire. In the 1960s, researchers William Masters and Virginia Johnson laid out four linear phases of the human response cycle: excitement, plateau, orgasm, and resolution. Later, Helen Kaplan Singer built on their theory, proposing that desire is what motivates sex—and that you can't get aroused at all without that piece of the puzzle. More recently, Dr. Rosemary Basson broke it down even further, suggesting that there are two different types of desire: spontaneous desire and responsive desire.

Spontaneous desire is often more present in the beginning of a relationship and can fade over time (in the relationship or even as one ages). Unlike spontaneous desire, which pretty much comes automatically, responsive desire requires some kind of stimulus—i.e. arousal—in order for desire to develop. For some, the arousal pathway can be short while others need to travel down a longer runway to get aroused. Laurie Mintz, PhD and certified sex therapist, draws the distinction that receptive desire "goes beyond the biological feelings of desire (horniness) and takes into account relational, social, cultural and contextual aspects of desire." Bonding, affection, romance and intimacy can trigger receptiveness for desire as can dirty talk, touch, and other forms of flirtation.

Unlike the spontaneous crowd who pretty much feel desire automatically, responsive types start off neutral to sex and require some kind of stimulus in order for desire to develop. It's very clear when a penis owner spontaneously gets an erection when their partner walks in the door. Vulva owners can be spontaneously turned on, but more often than not need to travel down a desire runway to get to arousal. Physical touch, affection, bonding, dirty talking, or romance can trigger their desire. Generally speaking, vulva owners are more likely to experience responsive desire, while penis owners more often experience spontaneous desire.

Sometimes, desire is more inward or self-focused. Maybe you want to put on a favorite pair of underwear that makes you feel really sexy, read some erotica, or think about the last time you were really turned on. Remember that desire doesn't always have to be about having sex with a partner. You can feel desire by yourself. You are a sexual being who deserves to be ready for sexual pleasure, regardless of your relationship status.

While the above is true for the majority of the population, it is important to note that some people are asexual meaning they do not typically experience sexual arousal.

Now that you understand desire and arousal, let's start working through the Sex IQ pillars to get smarter about sex.

Pillar #1: Embodiment

Can you think of a time when you allowed your mind to override a physical urge? Maybe you felt hungry at noon but pushed through and focused on work, and all of a sudden it was four o'clock and you still hadn't eaten. Or have you ever felt that you needed to go to the bathroom, but your mind kept you occupied until you could barely make it without having an accident?

Our bodies are always trying to tell us things—like whether we're in pain (and why) or if a certain movement brings up a memory (and why) or if we really want and need to be touched like this or like that (and why). Unfortunately, we too often ignore these cues. Even worse, this is considered normal in our culture. We place value on thoughts and ideas instead of our innate bodily wisdom. As a result, most of us exist primarily in our minds, feeling very disconnected from our bodies.

Even recently as we have learned more about the "mind-body connection," we still refer to it as a connection and not in a holistic way. In reality, the mind and body aren't separate. And they aren't merely connected. They're parts of the same whole.

Becoming embodied means that you are developing a new kind of awareness of your body that allows you to pick up on its cues. Instead of feeling like a brain that's walking around inside of a body, your brain and body become integrated, maintaining a constant two-way conversation. In essence, we need to remind our brains to listen to our bodies! This is an essential step toward reaching your pleasure potential.

The more present we are in our bodies, the more we can pay attention and tune in to the fact that we are becoming aroused, that something feels good to us, or that something doesn't feel right. We simply cannot fully feel and experience pleasure if we do not know how to pick up on these subtle cues.

Many of us feel that we are "in our heads" when we are having sex. We can barely feel what's happening in our bodies, never mind figure out whether or not we like it. We are too busy thinking instead of feeling. Our minds are filled with thoughts about what we might look and sound and smell like, all of the things we have to do later, or a conversation that we had with our partner earlier that night.

So there we are, naked with our partner with the intention of feeling good, and all we can do is worry about whether we're being too loud, how our body looks at this angle, and if our partner really wants to be having sex with us in the first place.

Clearly, this leaves no room for us to fully experience our body's sensations. If a certain position is painful, we just grin and bear it. We don't want to complain, or we think something is wrong with us. If we feel pleasure, we don't fully experience that, either. We're just going through the motions, lost in thought or maybe just trying to get off instead of being present in our pleasure. We're doing the things that are supposed to be the most pleasurable in the world, but we're putting all kinds of pressure on ourselves to orgasm or to make our partner orgasm. Where is the room here for authentic sexual connection?

When we focus on being more embodied during sex, it's a whole different ball game. Suddenly, we are in tune with everything that our bodies are experiencing. The skin on our partner's shoulders feels so soft, so we continue touching it. It makes us shiver when they drag their fingertips along our inner thighs, and we breathe into that sensation.

This attunement heightens our pleasure not just during sex, but in every moment of our lives in between and leading up to sexual experiences. Paying attention to our bodies is a daily practice. Now we notice that when our partner kisses us we are starting to become aroused. Or maybe we are aware of the fact that we started having sex too soon and need to slow down in order to become fully engaged and fully aroused.

Embodiment is not binary—we are not either embodied or not embodied. It is a continuum, and we will never be permanently, completely embodied. But becoming as embodied as you can is an important, pleasure-enhancing practice. The good news is that recognizing when you're not embodied counts as part of the practice. It may sound counterintuitive, but the more often you realize you're not embodied, the closer you're getting to being more embodied. You'll be able to feel more in your body and connect more deeply to your partner.

If you want to know what embodiment looks like, take a minute to watch young kids playing on a playground. Their minds and bodies aren't separate at all as they jump and run and leap and fly and fall with abandon.

It's no coincidence that kids are extremely sensitive to their bodies' sensations. They'll tell you right away when something hurts, or when something feels good. This is because they are listening to each and every cue from their bodies.

We are born this way, but we are conditioned away from our body's felt experiences. It's often around puberty when this all changes. Shoulders hunch, heads lower, and we begin to prioritize the opinions of others rather than our own feelings. For most of us, this never goes back. But our bodies have things that they want to say to us. As adults, we need to reopen that conversation.

Numbing—the Anti-Embodiment Practice

The practice of numbing messages from our bodies, emotions, and minds is pervasive in our culture, and it is the source of so much of our pain and suffering. When I talk about numbing, I am referring to anything that we do to distract ourselves from how we're really feeling. This is a way of taking ourselves out of the moment instead of being present and attuned.

We numb ourselves by eating food that doesn't make us feel good, shopping online, scrolling mindlessly on social media, drinking too much, getting high, or watching porn excessively—anything that distracts us from our emotions. We do these things hoping that they will make us feel good. And they do, for a moment, because they lead our bodies to release a quick hit of dopamine, a chemical messenger that plays an important role in the "reward center" of our brains.

Dopamine gives us a quick "high," but it's a fast burn, and then we quickly go back to baseline. And we are tricked into thinking that this is what pleasure really feels like. Dopamine also plays a role in motivation, so it encourages us to do whatever we can to get another hit of dopamine—often through activities that don't bring us true joy or fulfillment.

Think about how it feels when you click the "buy now" button. You get a quick hit of dopamine, and you feel good. You're happy with your purchase. But then you go back to baseline quickly, and you realize that you're not really satisfied. So, you click on another site and start adding more things that you don't really need to your cart. Does this sound familiar?

Numbing dampens our Sex IQ, keeping us from being embodied and attuned to what our partner is feeling. And the more we numb ourselves, the stronger those numbing muscles get. Over time, it becomes harder and harder to get back to the presence and embodiment that we need to experience pleasure.

The good news is that evolving our Sex IQ can help relieve our need to numb our body's messages. There are three essential practices that can help you become more embodied: mindful movement, meditation, and breath work.

Mindful Movement

Moving mindfully, while paying attention to the body and all of its sensations, helps us to become more embodied and restart that conversation between our brain and body. I'm not talking about mechanical exercises that we do with a goal in mind, though those are important for pillar #2, Health. Rather, mindful movement puts the focus on what we are feeling in our body. It helps us release tension and tune in to our body's signals.

Good options for mindful movement include yoga, dancing, martial arts, rock climbing, and taking slow walks without scrolling and while tuning in to all of your senses—anything that encourages you to be present in your body. As you engage in these activities, focus on what your body is feeling and experiencing. Tune in to what feels good and what doesn't. This will help you become more embodied and able to fully experience pleasure during sex and throughout your life.

Meditation

When we are mindful, we are fully in the moment and completely tuned in to our senses. This is the essence of embodiment. Meditation helps us tap into this powerful state because it is the practice of disengaging with our thoughts and allowing ourselves to simply be. When we meditate, thoughts do pop up, but when we practice letting them go without engaging with them, we gain the ability to be present in our body regardless of what is going on in our mind.

This can translate directly into sexual experiences. With a mindfulness meditation practice, you would be able to let go of the distracting thoughts that prevent you from being fully present and engaged. You would be able to tune in to your senses and experience more pleasure, even when those pesky thoughts arise.

I do my best to bookend my days by meditating once in the morning and then again at the end of the day. Even if I can't do it twice a day or if my morning mediation is only a few minutes, it still makes a huge difference. Two minutes of meditation is better than zero minutes. When we start our day with an established and consistent practice, it sets us up for success.

It doesn't matter what kind of meditation practice you choose or if you do it with the help of an app or any other tools. There are countless resources out there for you—check out my favorites in the back of the book. Taking a few minutes every day to get grounded and in touch with your body will help you become embodied and able to experience more and more pleasure.

Breath Work

Our breath is literally our life force, and besides keeping us alive, our breath can also shift us in or out of a state of stress, bring us into altered states of consciousness, and even bring us to orgasm. (More on this later.) The other interesting thing about our breath is that although it happens automatically without us thinking about it, we can also control it. When we control our breath; we can use it to do incredibly powerful things. One of those things is to connect with every part of our body.

When we want to feel less or when we feel pressure, we might subconsciously hold our breath. But becoming embodied means feeling *more.* We can use our breath to do this, too. Breath work is incredibly powerful in calming the nervous system to ease anxiety.

To start using the breath to become more embodied, simply focus on breathing deeper and longer, two of my favorite words when it comes to sex. See how high you can count on the inhale and then match it on the exhale or make your exhales are even longer. This will calm the body and help you feel more present.

As you continue to breathe, imagine that breath going all the way down to your pelvic floor. Give it a little squeeze on the inhale. Just say hello! This will open up the sexual energy fields that so many of us keep blocked off.

Remember that embodiment is a practice. None of us ever walks around fully embodied. But the more we sharpen our attunement to our body, the more we're able to call on these skills during sex. When we're distracted, we can go back to our senses and feel them more keenly. When we catch ourselves holding our breath, we can breathe deeply to feel more pleasure. And with more awareness of our bodily sensations in general, we are empowered to move toward those that are more pleasurable. This is precisely why embodiment is such an important part of your Sex IQ.

Embodiment Exercises

Body Scan Meditation

A body scan meditation is a great way to reconnect to your body and tune in to what it is feeling. To do this, sit comfortably or lie down, and close your eyes. Take a moment to just check in with your body. Where can you feel it touching the surface that you're sitting or lying on?

Now begin to focus on the breath entering your nose, filling your lungs, and going down to your belly. Imagine yourself expanding with each inhale and contracting with each exhale. If your mind wanders, just gently bring it back to the breath.

After a few minutes, direct your attention to your feet. Do you feel any sensations? Are they hot or cold or neither? Can you feel the texture of your socks or the floor beneath your heels? Now move on to your lower legs. Do you feel any tightness or tingling on your skin? What about in your muscles or bones? Whatever you feel is okay. There is no right or wrong.

When you're ready, move on to your upper legs. Notice anything you feel there. If you feel any tension, see if you can soften it. If not, that's okay. Just accept whatever you feel. Then move up to the pelvis. Notice any sensation in your hips, your buttocks, and your groin. Let go of any tension and see if you can sink deeper.

Then, as you continue breathing, move up to your stomach, then your chest, back, arms, wrists, hands, neck, and shoulders. Finally, move your awareness to your face. Are you clenching your jaw? Do you feel any tension in your temples? Try to allow yourself to soften.

Take a few more moments to breathe. Then take a moment to appreciate yourself for taking the time to reconnect with your body. When you are ready, open your eyes. Your body will likely feel more relaxed.

This is one of the best exercises to directly connect your body and mind and identify areas that are tense. Try it anytime you're feeling anxious or stressed, or do it as a daily practice. You can also do it quickly or stretch it out over twenty minutes. It's normal for emotions to come up. Pay attention to everything you are feeling physically and emotionally as a part of your embodiment practice.

When we can identify where we feel things like tension in our body, we are developing a skill that can translate to sex. Eventually it will become habitual, and during sex we will be more mindful of when we feel pleasure or pain. When we are more tuned in to what feels good and what doesn't, we can share that with a partner to experience even more pleasure.

4-7-8 Breathing

To practice 4-7-8 breathing, place one hand on your belly and the other on your chest. Count to four as you take a deep, slow breath into your belly. Hold your breath for seven counts. Breathe out for eight counts. Try to get all the air out of your lungs by the time you count to eight. Repeat three to seven times or until you feel calm, then take a few minutes to sit and feel the sensations in your body and mind before returning to your day.

Box Breathing

To try box breathing, sit with your back supported in a comfortable chair and your feet on the floor. Close your eyes and then breathe in through the nose while counting to four slowly, feeling the air enter into your lungs. Then hold the breath while counting slowly to four, trying not to clamp your mouth or nose shut, and slowly exhale for four seconds. Repeat this at least three times.

Try pausing a few times throughout the day and breathing like this for just a few minutes. This will help you become more present and mindful and connected to your body. Over time, you will likely start to notice moments during the day when your breathing becomes shallow, and you'll have a chance to correct yourself. This awareness is a huge step toward becoming more embodied. During sex, if you sense yourself becoming anxious or distracted, you can stop and breathe deeply. It will help you become more present and embodied almost immediately.

Pillar #2: Health

When I talk about health, I don't mean having a six-pack or a body that looks any one particular way. I'm referring to your vitality, the ease with which blood flows through your veins, the delicate balance of your hormones, the functionality of your cells and organs, and the exact makeup of your microbiome. All of these things affect your sexual experiences, probably in ways that you've never realized. Everything that you put into your body—from food to medicines—impacts your health in some way and has a direct impact on your pleasure, too.

To get a clearer understanding of how your health is impacting your sexual wellness, I recommend checking to see if you are up-to-date on all of your health screenings and dental checkups. Yes, even the health of your teeth and gums can impact your pleasure. When inflammation in the gums leads to more serious conditions like gingivitis or periodontitis, it increases your risk of tooth decay, cardiovascular disease, stroke, and various types of cancer. All of these issues directly impact your sexual health. If that's not a good reason to floss, I don't know what is.

To prioritize your health, the nonnegotiables are: good nutrition, exercise (cardio and weights), adequate sleep, time in nature, and quality social connections. These all impact your sexuality. For example, eating a lot of foods that are high in saturated fats and rarely moving your body can inhibit blood flow, making it more difficult for you to become aroused. When we're not feeling healthy, we're often sluggish and fatigued. This can keep us from feeling confident and energized, preventing us from wanting to have sex.

Your mental health, meaning your psychological and emotional well-being, also plays a big role in your ability to access pleasure. If you struggle with anxiety, for example, it won't just magically disappear in the bedroom. And if you're suffering from depression, it can directly impact your ability to become aroused. Trauma, which I'll discuss in great detail later, can also prevent you from enjoying sex. You'll never reach your pleasure potential if you're not monitoring your mental health and taking necessary steps to improve, whether that's through therapy, medications, or simply taking more time for self-care. If you're not motivated to do it for any other reason, do it for the sake of your sex life!

The Sex IQ pillars all work together. You might notice that the more in tune you are with your body, the more motivated you'll be to start taking care of your health. This is a great side effect of embodiment. When we tune in and start to listen to our body's cues, it becomes easier to get to the root cause of our pain and heal.

I can't talk about the connection between sex and health without bringing up the very real possibility of contracting a sexually transmitted infection (STI) or disease (STD). You can get an STI or STD from most sex acts. The only way to completely avoid this is abstinence, but that's not exactly what this book is about. So, I am here to encourage you to practice safe, smart sex. Use condoms and dental dams, get tested regularly, talk to your partners to make sure they're getting tested, and only engage in sex acts with partners you trust.

If you do contract an STI or STD, please know that it's very common, and it does not mean that your sex life is over. Be honest with your partners, be careful about practicing safe sex, and educate yourself about how to manage the symptoms and avoid spreading it to others.

Outside of STDs and STIs, there are three aspects of your physical health that have the greatest impact on your sexual health. They are: your hormones, your medications, and your gut.

Hormones

We tend to think of hormones primarily when it comes to menstruation and pregnancy, but they impact your desire and arousal in many other ways. Since vulva owners' hormones fluctuate throughout the month, their sexual desire ebbs and flows constantly. But the importance of hormones when it comes to sexual health for both penis and vulva owners cannot be overstated. The sooner we start paying attention to our hormone levels, the more control we will have over our arousal and pleasure.

Because many different hormones work together in a delicate balance, even small changes in certain hormone levels can dramatically impact your health and specifically your sexual health. The good news is that to a great extent, you can control this. It is possible to take your hormones into your own hands and make necessary changes.

Some of the most important ways to balance your hormones are to get proper nutrition, especially adequate protein, reduce sugar consumption, exercise regularly, and get enough sleep. If you take these steps, you really might start to see a difference in your sexual health.

Any number of hormones can affect our sexual health, but here I'll focus on the ones that we typically think of when we think about our sexual health. These are appropriately called sex hormones: estrogen, progesterone, and testosterone.

Estrogen: Estrogen is the main sex hormone in vulva owners, and it is produced by the ovaries. Between puberty and menopause, estrogen regulates the menstrual cycle and plays an important role in the urinary tract, cardiovascular system, musculoskeletal system, bones, breasts, skin, hair, mucous membranes, pelvic muscles, and brain. So, it's kind of important.

In menstruating vulva owners, levels of estrogen rise and fall throughout the menstrual cycle. Since estrogen increases vaginal lubrication and sexual desire, it makes sense that those things ebb and flow throughout the month, too. If you're a vulva owner who's not always in the mood to have sex or doesn't always have the same amount of lubrication, rest assured that this is completely normal. It's not you—it's your estrogen!

Sadly, in our disembodied culture, many vulva owners have fallen out of sync with their cycles. It is incredibly empowering for vulva owners to get back in touch with the natural wisdom of their bodies and gain familiarity with their cycles. This will help you learn so much invaluable information about your sexual desire and arousal.

Because of cycling hormones, vulva owners often experience higher levels of sexual desire around the time of ovulation (midcycle). Some even report experiencing more satisfaction from an orgasm at around this time. After ovulation, most vulva owners experience a dip in sexual desire. Of course, this isn't true for everyone. If you have a period, it's useful to track your desire with your cycle and see how your hormones are affecting you.

As vulva owners approach menopause, their estrogen levels naturally drop. For many, this leads to struggles with a lack of desire and vaginal dryness, but it does not have to be this way. It is possible to have a very hot and satisfying sex life during perimenopause and after menopause.

At this time of life, the mental aspects of desire can become even more important. This alone (plus plenty of lube, of course) can really help. I also encourage you to find a healthcare provider who specializes in women's hormone health and can talk to you about whether hormone replacement therapy or other treatments might be appropriate and helpful. This can help with arousal and desire, as well as many other symptoms of menopause.

Penis owners, did you know that you have estrogen in your bodies, too? Your testes and brains produce it. When penis owners produce too much estrogen, it can slow down sperm production and cause erectile dysfunction. Interestingly, when penis owners produce too little estrogen, it can lead to many of the same symptoms.

Today it's very common for both penis and vulva owners to have high estrogen levels, often because of exposure to xenoestrogens, which are chemicals in our environment that mimic estrogen in our bodies. Examples of xenoestrogens include bisphenol A (BPA) and phthalates, both of which are present in certain types of plastics. Phthalates are also in many common personal care products, from soaps to lotions to shampoos. If you don't already, start looking at labels and minimizing your use of these items as much as possible, in addition to the other ways of balancing hormones.

Progesterone: In vulva owners, the body makes progesterone to help support a potential pregnancy after ovulation has occurred. If the egg isn't fertilized, progesterone levels drop, leading to menstruation. If the egg is fertilized, the body continues to produce progesterone to support the pregnancy. Progesterone also helps trigger lactation once the baby is born.

The relationship between your libido and progesterone levels is not black-and-white. Some studies find that higher progesterone increases sex drive, while other studies show that the opposite is true. This may be because some bodies are more sensitive to hormones than others. Or it could be because these studies don't look at the all-important balance between progesterone and estrogen.

In fact, your progesterone levels themselves are less important than how they relate to your estrogen levels. Most people have the strongest libido when there is a healthy ratio of estrogen to progesterone. In addition to reduced sexual desire, symptoms of an estrogen and progesterone imbalance include irregular menstruation, infertility, weight gain, fatigue, anxiety, and depression. Don't let anyone tell you that these symptoms are in your head! Get your hormone levels tested and begin to work toward achieving hormonal balance.

Penis owners have progesterone, too. In fact, progesterone is a building block of testosterone. Just like in vulva owners, it is important for penis owners to have the right balance between estrogen and progesterone. When this balance is off, penis owners can suffer from anxiety, erectile dysfunction, fatigue, prostate enlargement, a higher risk of prostate cancer, and low libido.

Because testosterone is made in part from progesterone, low levels of progesterone lead to low levels of testosterone, our last and perhaps most important sex hormone.

Testosterone: Testosterone is the main sex hormone in penis owners, but vulva owners have testosterone, too. In fact, the bodies of vulva owners use testosterone to make estrogen. Testosterone plays an important role in the libidos of both penis and vulva owners, as well as in their bone and muscle health and their mood.

Like estrogen, testosterone levels drop in vulva owners during menopause. This can lead to low libido and vaginal dryness. In penis owners, low levels of testosterone can lead to reduced sexual desire, as well as erectile dysfunction and reduced sperm count. Again, I recommend talking to your doctor about hormone replacement therapy, which can help with these issues.

Remember that lifestyle changes can make a big impact here. Unless there is a deeper issue at play, the best ways to achieve hormonal balance are by eating a healthy diet, exercising, reducing stress levels, and getting enough sleep. Once you start eating healthier, you really might get your erections back. And more sleep might actually equal more vaginal lubrication. But it is very possible to be doing all of these things right and still have imbalanced hormones, which leads me to my next topic...

Medications

Taking the medications that you need is an essential part of being healthy. However, it's important to know that many prescription medications do affect our sexual health. They can lower our libidos and reduce our ability to sustain erections, become lubricated during sex, and even orgasm. These are called sexual side effects. Doctors sometimes mention them briefly when prescribing a medication, or you might see them buried in a long list of possible side effects on your medication's label, but I think that they deserve a lot more attention than that.

I would never tell you to not take a medication that you need. But talk to your doctor about the medicines you are taking and any sexual side effects that you may be experiencing. Sometimes there are alternatives or other ways of counteracting these effects that can be very helpful.

One major class of drugs that often leads to sexual side effects is antidepressants. In particular, selective serotonin reuptake inhibitors (SSRIs) commonly lead to a delayed or absent orgasm, meaning it takes a long time to have an orgasm or you can't have one at all. This can be very frustrating for people who take these medications and finally start to feel desire again, only to be unable to orgasm. If this is you, don't lose hope. There are many different medications out there, and some people experience side effects with some SSRIs but not others. Sometimes a switch from one SSRI to another will help you orgasm again.

In addition, heart and blood pressure medications; opioids; and statins, which are used to lower cholesterol, can all cause sexual side effects. It is interesting to consider the role of statins in particular, as testosterone is made from cholesterol, and these medications have been shown to reduce testosterone along with cholesterol levels. Everything in our bodies is connected!

This brings me finally to birth control pills (and other forms of hormonal birth control like some IUDs—the copper IUD does not have hormones), which affect our sexual health probably more than any other medication. Most forms of hormonal birth control are made with synthetic forms of estrogen and progesterone that interfere with the process that leads to ovulation and menstruation. This helps you avoid pregnancy. It's wonderful for vulva owners to be in control of their bodies this way.

You knew there was a "but" coming, right? Unfortunately, this control over our reproductive systems comes with a price, in the form of some major hormonal havoc. Birth control pills can lower testosterone levels, which reduces libido. The scariest part is that these levels typically don't bounce back after going off the pill. This long-term reduction in testosterone can lead to a variety of problems, including weakened muscles and bones and ongoing sexual side effects.

The birth control pill can also mess with your neurotransmitter levels; in particular the neurotransmitter serotonin, which controls your mood, is responsible for feelings of happiness, and plays a big role in sexual desire. Ugh! This explains why vulva owners who are on the pill are more likely to start taking an SSRI, which often compounds these sexual side effects. So, the pill makes you feel depressed with low desire, you take an SSRI to feel better, and suddenly your desire drops even lower and you can't have an orgasm. Not a great formula for a satisfying sex life.

But here's where it gets really interesting. We are on the forefront of learning about all of the ways that our hormones affect us. This growing body of research shows that estrogen plays a big role not only in your desire and arousal, but also in your choice of sexual partner.

During a standard menstrual cycle, when estrogen levels go up they increase a vulva owner's sexual desire—but not a desire for just anyone. Estrogen itself increases desire for partners whose features indicate that they have high levels of testosterone and can therefore provide healthy genetic material for children. (These studies were obviously done on cisgender, heterosexual couples. With more research, it will be fascinating to learn more about how estrogen affects sexual desire and partner selection in other types of couples.)

The birth control pill, however, keeps estrogen at a low, steady level throughout the month. Studies have shown that this has a direct impact on who those people taking the pill are sexually attracted to and even their choice of partners.

So, you may be wondering, what happens when they stop taking the pill?

Researchers spoke to two groups of vulva owners about the quality of their relationships. The first group chose their partners when they were on the pill, and the second chose their partners when they were not on the pill. The group who chose their partner while on the pill were now less sexually attracted to their partners! They also reported less sexual arousal in response to their partners, and less sexual adventurousness than the second group. Further studies have shown similar results.

Of course, this is not a problem for everyone. I'm certain that many vulva owners who take birth control pills have fully satisfying relationships and sex lives. But many are unaware of the side effects. If you are struggling with any aspect of your sexual health, it is worth putting all of the medications that you are taking on the table. Consider what side effects they might be causing and if it's worth looking at alternatives. Understanding all of these factors is important to improving your Sex IQ.

The Gut

Like hormones, the gut is an emerging area of research, and one that I am obsessed with. We are going to be learning so much more over the next few years about all of the ways that the bacteria in our guts impact different aspects of our health and well-being.

For now, let's focus on how the gut affects our sex hormones. Oh, did you not know that was a thing? The gut bacteria and the substances they produce actually impact the levels of sex hormones circulating in the body. At the same time, hormones regulate the diversity of the gut biome, or the population of natural bacteria in our gut. A highly diverse gut biome with many different species of bacteria is a major marker of good health.

In other words, your hormones and gut biome each affect each other in a bidirectional system. Studies show that men who suffer from erectile dysfunction have less microbial diversity than men without erectile dysfunction. Some researchers are even looking into probiotics as a way of treating erectile dysfunction.

The best ways to create a healthy, diverse gut biome are to exercise, eat a variety of plant foods including plenty of fiber, and avoid antibiotics as much as possible. We have known since the 1980s that taking antibiotics, which kill off certain species of gut bacteria, can lead to changes in estrogen levels. You really might start eating more fiber or taking a high-quality probiotic and notice an increase in your desire and arousal. It's certainly worth a try.

The birth control pill also has an impact on your gut health. Dr. Jolene Brighten, a naturopathic physician, explains that birth control pills can lead to leaky gut (a permeable intestinal wall that can cause proteins and other waste to be released into your system), yeast overgrowth, decreased microbial diversity, and altered gut mobility, which can lead to small intestinal bacterial overgrowth (SIBO). All of this wreaks further havoc on your sex hormones, impacting your libido and your ability to become erect and lubricated.

There are many nonhormonal birth control options, including condoms, copper IUDs, the sponge, and tracking your cycles. Consult with your doctor to make the best decisions for you and your body.

Was it Hippocrates who said that all great sex starts in the gut? I might have that wrong, but it is true that having a healthy gut can help you balance your sex hormones and become healthier for better sex and higher Sex IQ. So, clean up the diet, hit the gym, and then hit the sheets if you want to take your sex life to the next level.

Pillar #3: Collaboration

Part of who you are as a sexual being is how you relate to your partner(s) and work with them to co-create meaningful and fulfilling intimate and sexual experiences. Many of the people I talk to crave intimacy and closeness and not just sex. It takes intentional collaboration to create a relationship that includes both.

Many people think they're already collaborating when it comes to sex. After all, it takes two to tango. But the pattern I see the most often is that they don't talk about their sex life, assume their partner should know how to please them, and aren't invested in each other's pleasure. Then they fall into the trap of failing to prioritize their relationship over other things like work and kids. They start feeling frustrated about their partner not pleasing them. They're not connecting energetically and checking in with each other often. Eventually, resentment builds and their sex life suffers. I can't tell you how common this cycle is and how easy it is to avoid it with intentional collaboration.

The absolute most important and effective tool to collaborate well is consistent and honest communication. I always say that communication is a form of lubrication because, like lube, it is an absolute must for enhancing sexual satisfaction. It's so important that it has its own chapter later in the book, where you'll find tips and scripts to help you find the right time, words, and ways to communicate about sex. Here, I'd like to focus on two aspects of sexual collaboration that are often overlooked: sexual energy and polarity.

Sexual Energy

Sex and relationships are obviously all about connection. When you are intimately connected to someone, the energy that you bring to that relationship both in and out of the bedroom is all-important. Everything is energy. Cyndi Dale, author of *The Subtle Body*, explains, "The human body is a complex energetic system, composed of hundreds of energetic subsystems."

You cannot see energy, but you can feel it. Sexual energy is the feelings of arousal in your body. Of course, becoming more embodied helps you tune in to your sexual energy.

When you are deeply connected, you can also feel your partner's sexual energy. The best ways to do this are through breath, touch, and looking into each other's eyes. When you look into your partner's eyes, tune in to how it makes you feel. You are connecting with their energy. This energetic connection is a huge part of creating intimacy.

In many relationships, conflict arises when one partner feels the other isn't making time for them. The real problem here is that they don't feel connected. And when partners are disconnected energetically, the sex and overall relationship really suffers.

Of course, it's important to make time for your partner, but sustaining a connection doesn't always require a lot of time. When it's not possible to spend a lot of time together, I recommend taking just a few minutes each day to connect with your partner's energy.

Someone with a vulva came to me complaining that she didn't have enough sex with her partner and felt that they were very disconnected. I advised her to create a practice of breathing with her partner. Every day when she got home from work, she took a few minutes to look into her eyes and breathe deeply without talking. If this seems too out of reach or you can't imagine gazing into your partner's eyes like this, there's also a lot of power in a simple thirty-second hug. In the case of this couple, this practice made them feel more energetically connected and intimate. After some time, this energetic connection translated to the bedroom, where they were more attuned and sensitive to each other's verbal and nonverbal cues.

Sexual Polarity

Our bodies crave a partner with energy that is complementary to ours. To create the hottest sex, this means opposite or opposing energies. Polarity is the attraction of opposites. Think of a battery with a positive charge on one end and a negative charge on the other. When the opposites connect, it creates an electric charge.

It's important to understand opposing energy particularly when you're trying to enhance your sexual connection. It can also help you understand your arousal. To have hotter sex with more magnetism and electricity, we need to increase the extremity of those opposites. The more opposing your energy is from your partner's, the more attracted you will be.

When we talk about sexual polarity, we refer to opposite energies as masculine and feminine, but each of us contains both types of energy, and this is not about the gender binary. This is a tricky concept, but it has really helped me understand sexual energies. When I've done podcasts on this subject, especially with coach John Wineland, they've been the most listened to episodes of the year. The challenge is that many people (understandably) get caught up in the labels of masculine and feminine. We typically associate any discussion of masculine and feminine with gender or sexual orientation. But for this conversation, I ask you to consider masculine and feminine energies as inherent in all of us. Even in same-sex relationships there is a presence of masculine and feminine energies. Through this lens we can use them as tools to help us understand attraction and arousal in relation to our partners. This is more of a theory than an exact science, but my goal is to help you think differently about energy and desire.

Every vulva and penis owner has a unique combination of masculine and feminine energies. In fact, considering these energies is a good way of understanding the full spectrum of gender identity and expression. If the terms "masculine" and "feminine" don't work for you, you can try replacing them with "yin" and "yang"—a symbol of opposite but interconnected forces.

Masculine sexual energy is mission-driven, decisive, initiative, and structured, while feminine sexual energy is freer and more open, tender, intuitive, and creative. Typically, one partner prefers to show up in one type of energy during sexual experiences. Or maybe you like to shift between masculine and feminine energies. Sometimes your energy is more masculine, and other times it's more feminine. That's awesome, too, and this is where collaboration comes in. You and your partner can play around by animating different sides of yourselves, leaning into opposite energies to increase your electric charge.

When it comes to sex, masculine energy typically shows up as leading and initiating, while feminine energy is more receptive. The partner with the masculine energy makes the plans, sets the direction for the evening, and tells the partner what is going to happen, while keeping their best interests in mind. The partner with feminine energy follows and accepts their partner's plans, ultimately submitting to them. To put it simply, one partner leads so the other can follow.

I've learned that a key component of my arousal is leaning into my feminine energy. For me, that's the spark that really gets the sex going! During the day when I'm working, I'm typically in my masculine energy. If I've been in meetings all day focusing on my mission and I know I want to have sex with my partner that night, I take some time to intentionally shift my energy by grounding myself, stretching, and doing some breath work. Since our systems are interconnected, this allows my partner to lean into their masculine energy. The energy you exude typically evokes the opposite in your partner.

So, when my partner is really in his masculine energy, he is responsible, clear, capable, and stable. He is taking charge, making plans, and has a direction. This allows me to feel more of my feminine energy. When he says, "I made a reservation at seven on Thursday at our favorite sushi place. I'll pick you up," this directness, prior planning, and confidence allows me to let go and lean into my feelings of excitement for the evening and my desire to nurture him and our connection. I can relax and be present and embodied. The feminine is a receiving energy that brings lightness and curiosity to the moment, allowing me to notice and point out a beautiful sunset or, as cheesy as it sounds, stop and smell the roses.

When I don't focus on being in my feminine energy, I'm directing things with a harder edge. I'm less receptive to his touch because I'm in less of a receiving mode. It's all very nuanced, but I notice in these moments that we don't get along as well. We're like two positive ends of a battery with no charge.

Of course, this also applies to same-sex relationships. Someone has to lead with their masculine energy and someone has to lean into their feminine energy. Many vulva owners like stepping up and taking initiative instead. This is about masculine and feminine, not vulva and penis. It's a cycle of polarity, and it's another way of understanding and enhancing attraction and desire.

When partners have similar sexual energies, their connection feels more platonic, without that sexual charge. This can happen in long-term relationships when partners spend all of their time together doing the same predictable activities with no variety, novelty, or surprise. To sustain sexual chemistry, it's important to work together to intentionally maintain polarity.

It can be fun to switch it up and have the partner who doesn't normally initiate sex summon their masculine energy, take charge, and initiate. Even better, this partner could make the plans for the entire evening, including during sex. This would give the other partner a chance to explore their feminine energy.

For example, I spoke to a couple, Jen and Dori, who like to take turns initiating and receiving. Sometimes Jen wants to be dominated or directed, and other times Dori wants to lie back, relinquish control, and just receive. They both enjoy role-playing by dressing up as different genders and playing authority figures. This allows for their yin and yang to be expressed in various ways.

This tension of opposites can be created in a million different ways, but it does take an awareness of the necessity for purposeful decisiveness to be met with eager receptivity.

Start to tune in and feel when you are in your masculine or feminine energy. It will likely shift a bit throughout the day depending on what you're doing. Just notice. Then when you are with your partner, you can lean into the energy that will create more polarity between the two of you.

To explore polarity, take turns with your partner initiating sex. Perhaps you agree that each one of you will initiate once a week or month. The partner with the "masculine energy" will pick the night, set the plans, and take control in the bedroom. The other partner agrees to participate in the evening while being mindful of their urges to take the lead or go off course. By relinquishing control and allowing your partner to lead, you'll find yourself letting go and leaning more into your feminine energy.

Exercise—Tantric Breathing

A powerful way to connect and exchange sexual energy is through breath work. Tantric breath work in particular is not about having an orgasm that lasts all day. It is a way to activate sexual energy between partners, building intimacy and magnetism.

To try this, sit facing each other, ideally with one partner sitting on the other's lap with the legs wrapped around their waist. The "base" partner is the partner choosing to lead from their masculine energy, either for this one exercise or more consistently. They are providing the structure. The partner sitting on top is the one with the feminine energy of receiving. Try switching up who sits on the other's lap to evoke different types of sexual energy.

Once you are in position, you can simply look into each other's eyes and breathe. After a few minutes, your breath will sync up on its own. If you stop here, you will feel deeply connected. But to take this a step further, begin to move together, swaying your hips from side to side, finding a rhythm together. This activates your sexual energy, with the base partner giving their energy to the receptive partner on top. You will likely be shocked by the sensation of the energy moving between you and how powerful it is.

This is a great practice for any couple that is curious about exchanging sexual energy. It can also be especially helpful for partners who feel that they have lost the spark in their relationship. It only takes a few minutes and can lead to profound results.

Pillar #4: Self-Knowledge

Earlier, we discussed desire and how it manifests physically through arousal. But desire can also start to build (or not) long before you're in the bedroom—even before you see your partner. There are countless environmental, physical, and psychological factors that can help us feel desire or that can block us from feeling it.

Do you know what yours are?

When it comes to sex, self-knowledge is about understanding your arousal patterns and exactly what you need in order to feel desire. Over the years, I have learned all of the factors that have to come into play for me to be in the mood for sex. I know that I have to feel connected to my partner. I need to have a conversation first. I need to feel safe. I need to be with a partner who is attentive to my needs. Just paying attention and knowing this has helped me navigate my sex life more authentically and openly.

It's important to know what in your environment will enhance or detract from your pleasure. In Emily Nagoski's book, *Come as You Are*, she explains the concept of contextual sexual desire, when circumstances and the environment impact our ability to feel sexual desire. I know that when the air conditioner is on full blast, it feels as though my blood flow freezes up and any sexual energy I previously had is now being spent trying to keep me warm. Some other common desire detractors are hearing the kids in the next room, a loud TV, having just eaten a big meal, clutter all over the bedroom, and on and on.

As you begin to learn about what does and doesn't do it for you, you can leverage your environment and your schedule to prime your brain and body for sexual pleasure. This will make it much easier for you to feel desire and become aroused when the time comes.

This is one reason that I often recommend scheduling sex. So many people assume that scheduling sex is boring or sad or a sign that their sex life is dead in the water, but it can actually be really hot, partly because it gives you time to create the ideal conditions for you to build your desire. This will help you work with your brain and body to kick-start your desire and arousal process instead of fighting against it.

Let's say you and your partner plan ahead to have sex on Saturday night. You can prepare everything in advance to increase your chances of being in the mood. Simply thinking about the fact that you're going to have sex later in the week and how good it will feel can help you build your desire. But to really prime the pump (so to speak), take it a step further. Maybe you can plan for the kids to sleep over at Grandma's house that night. Or maybe you can set the scene—light a fire, put some soft new sheets on the bed, play some nice music—whatever sounds sensual and pleasurable to you.

Or maybe you can take some time earlier that day to relax and experience other types of pleasure—take a bubble bath, indulge in a nap, or slowly and luxuriously massage your body with lotion after getting out of the shower. Who knows? Maybe you want to watch some porn before your date to get yourself excited.

The idea is to know exactly what you need to do to get yourself in the mood so you can intentionally create the ideal circumstances to maximize your pleasure. Pleasure compounds and makes it easier to give and receive. Pleasure begets pleasure!

Your Desire Inventory

Intentionally building desire is so important, yet many of us have no idea which factors help us feel erotic desire and which ones block it. We just know when we're feeling it and when we're not. This exercise will help you begin to identify the keys to unlock your personal desire.

Answer each of the questions below with a number on a scale of one to ten based on how important they are to building your desire—one being completely unimportant and ten being extremely important. Don't rank them—simply give them each a score.

How important is the following for you to get excited for sex with your partner?

- to connect with my partner emotionally, through spending time together and sharing conversation, before I can get excited for sex with them.
- to share something stimulating with someone, like a delicious meal, an interesting movie, or a physical activity, before I can get excited for sex with them.
- to have my partner flirt with me before I can get excited for sex with them.
- that my partner has dressed up and taken the time to look nice for me before I can get excited for sex with them.
- that I've dressed up for my partner and feel confident in my appearance before I can get excited for sex with them.
- to watch sexy media, like porn or a hot movie, before I can get excited to have sex with my partner.
- to feel safe and comfortable with someone before I can get excited for sex with them.
- to have given or received gifts (e.g., flowers, lingerie, toys, etc.) as a precursor to having sex with my partner.
- to role-play prior to and during a sexual encounter.
- to have mystery about the evening before having sex with my partner.

Now, look at your high scores, particularly any factors that you scored a five or above. Then try applying these conditions to your sexual encounters.

For example, let's say that your highest score was for sharing a stimulating experience with someone before having sex with them. Then you can't expect to feel erotic desire after spending the night chilling on the couch watching TV! Instead, ask yourself what kind of stimulating activity will give you the greatest possible boost in desire.

To figure this out, ask yourself when you have felt the most turned on. Maybe you always want to have sex right after you work out with your partner because you're super turned on when you're both sweaty and your blood is pumping, and this has led to amazing sex in the past. Great! Start exploring new physical activities that you can try together to enhance your desire even more. There's a biological component to this, as well. We release feel-good hormones when we exercise, which stimulates blood flow and helps with arousal.

You can apply this same type of logic to your future sexual encounters based on your own high scores.

If there are some examples above that you've never tried, now's the time to start experimenting with them and find out whether or not they boost your desire. I recommend that you share your results with your partner if you have one. Better yet, ask them to take the desire inventory and then compare answers so you better understand each other and can help facilitate an environment of arousal for both of you.

This is great information to communicate with your future partners, too, or to use to enhance your solo sex, something we'll discuss in much greater detail later. Please note that even if you ranked high on a particular point or points, that doesn't mean that you'll require all of these elements to be in place every single time you have sex. Just knowing your desire inventory is enough to help you boost your pleasure.

Core Desires

Taking this a step further, you can gain self-knowledge by identifying your core desires, a term I learned from Celeste Hirschman and Danielle Harel, sex educators and the authors of the book *Coming Together*, who built on the work of Jack Morin, another expert in eroticism. Your core desires are the specific feelings you want to experience during sex.

You don't choose your core desires. They are the result of your lived experience, usually stemming from moments in your childhood. Experts consider them our brain's attempts to heal childhood wounds, which—let's face it—we all have, even if our childhoods seemed perfect. In his seminal work, *The Erotic Mind*, Morin claims that at some point in childhood, something good or bad triggers a sexual response, and that experience lays the foundation for the specific feelings we require to be sexually present. These feelings are our core desires.

Sometimes, our core desires harken back to an unfulfilled childhood need. Maybe there was a certain emotion or feeling that we wanted to experience and didn't get when we were children. As adults, this can become the feeling that we most want to experience during sex, such as to be adored, worshipped, wanted, naughty, or to be the center of attention. These are feelings, not specific scenarios. There is an endless list of feelings that awaken and heighten your arousal.

Until you identify your core desires, your sexual satisfaction will be somewhat limited. Think of it as a sexual thirst that you can't quite quench. When you become familiar with your core desires, however, you can approach any sexual situation knowing exactly what feelings will make you feel the most nourished and fulfilled.

Because most of us have never reflected on our core desires, we tend to walk into new sexual situations like we're rolling the dice—*I hope I like this! I guess we'll find out.* At the same time, we enter familiar yet unsatisfying sexual situations feeling somewhat resigned—*Oh, this again.* But you actually have a say in this equation. When you know your core desires and what you're solving for, the rest of the factors are usually pretty easy to fill in. You can intentionally create sexual scenarios that help you experience the feeling you most want during sex.

Having an orgasm is one thing. Walking away from a sexual encounter feeling truly satisfied is another. In order to achieve the latter, you must develop a deep understanding of yourself as a sexual being.

Start by asking yourself this: What comes to mind when you think about the hottest sexual moment you've ever had, or that you've ever imagined? It doesn't have to be an elaborate scene or a full-fledged fantasy. You can learn a lot about yourself by identifying even the smallest, seemingly insignificant things that turned you on, especially if you can find a pattern among these moments. These patterns are clues to your core desires.

Once you identify these moments, go a little deeper and ask yourself: In that real or imagined moment, how did you feel emotionally? Did you feel adored or powerful or something that might surprise you, like humiliated or degraded? These feelings that turn you on the most tend to be your core desires. Your fantasies or most exciting sexual moments are ways of experiencing your core desires.

To get your wheels turning, here are some examples of fantasies and how they connect to core desires:

If you get turned on by the idea of having sex in public, it could mean that your core desire is for you to be so wanted that your partner can't wait another minute and will have sex with you anywhere. Or it could mean that you want to feel a little naughty or transgressive, like you're getting away with something.

If you fantasize about your partner surprising you with a decadent meal at your favorite five-star restaurant, you might have a core desire of being cared for or seen and known. It took a lot of effort to plan the dinner, and they knew your favorite restaurant, which made you feel loved and nurtured. Or you might have a core desire to be pampered—for someone to be willing to go to great lengths to court you.

If you're a penis owner who gets really turned on by the idea of ejaculating on your partner's face, you may have a core desire of being fully accepted. If this person will take your semen on their face, they'll let you do anything. This could also signal a core desire around feeling messy or a little dirty. Or it might be about being in control without limits.

Core desires are not right or wrong. They just are. And getting to know yours will dramatically shift your Sex IQ and your sexual satisfaction.

Your self-knowledge also includes everything that you've learned about yourself while growing in the other pillars. Maybe you realize that you haven't exercised in a while and that's why you haven't been in the mood for sex, or that a medication is keeping you from becoming aroused, or that your relationship has lost its spark because of a lack of polarity. These are huge steps toward understanding where you are right now as a sexual person. This knowledge also gives you the power to find workarounds so you can start having better sex no matter where you are starting from.

There are few things in life that are more important than your relationship with yourself, and to enhance that relationship you need self-awareness. Throughout this book, you are going to find tools to help you dramatically grow your self-awareness during mindful masturbation, open communication with your partner(s), and a full exploration of your core desires.

Before I started this work, I never would have been able to

tell a partner how I wanted to be touched or what turned me on—because I didn't even know! If that's where you are right now, that's okay. My goal is to help you continue getting to know yourself better as a uniquely sexual person who owns their own pleasure.

Once we get to know ourselves, however, there is another important step, which takes us to our next and final pillar.

Pillar #5: Self-Acceptance

In order to truly experience pleasure, we must accept and love and find confidence in all aspects of ourselves, including our past mistakes, our bodies, our needs, our sexual histories, our skills as a lover, where we are in our sexual journey, and our unique wants and desires. We also must accept everything that we've learned about ourselves by exploring the other pillars. You have control over many of these things, and once you accept them, you can take the necessary steps to create change.

Accepting ourselves is one of the hardest things for many of us to do. From the media's depiction of beauty norms to social media's filtered images, it's extremely common to compare ourselves to others and feel that we come up short. It takes consistent effort to learn to accept and love ourselves as we are.

Unfortunately, insecurities around sex are extremely common. I doubt that there is one person reading this that does not feel insecure about some aspect of their sexual skills. I hope that it's comforting to know that many of us feel this way, even those people who society would consider to be the most sexually desirable.

Our confidence, or lack thereof, in other areas of our life can also affect our sexual confidence. So, really accepting yourself sexually means accepting all parts of your life.

Often, growing our self-awareness pillar helps us accept ourselves. We sometimes see this in vulva owners who have a sexual confidence that comes with age. They know themselves and what feels good. Even though their bodies have changed, they have the value of wisdom and experience.

I'm not suggesting that you are going to read this and then suddenly start believing that every part of you is perfect. But practicing self-compassion can help you go a long way toward accepting who you are right now. This is a practice of reminding yourself that even the parts of you that you may not like the most are still lovable and worthy and deserving of pleasure.

An important part of practicing self-compassion is monitoring your self-talk, or the narrative that is constantly going in your head. So many of us are not even conscious of how many times a day we think hateful, critical thoughts about ourselves. When we're constantly saying negative things to ourselves, it keeps us from wanting to be intimate and let someone else in.

Becoming aware of this is an important first step, and then you can consciously begin changing these thoughts. Every time you catch yourself thinking a negative thought about yourself, neutralize it with an affirmation. Experiment and find one that feels authentic and empowering to you. Try, "I accept my body. It is deserving of pleasure and love."

You can also practice appreciating parts of your body. Think about all of the things that your body does for you, especially the parts that you may feel insecure about. Then thank them—"Thank you to my thighs for giving me the strength to climb." When we connect to the parts we are critical of and appreciate how we use them functionally, it can help us learn to accept them.

Here's the thing that most people don't realize—sexual confidence doesn't come from being perfect, having lots of sexual experience, or from looking the way that society tells us is hot. It doesn't come from having a huge penis or knowing how to make your partner orgasm in thirty seconds. It comes from a sense of neutrality—not judging yourself in a positive or negative light. Just living in harmony with yourself. This is self-acceptance.

★★★

Whenever I find that I haven't been in the mood for sex or that something is off in the bedroom, I run through the Sex IQ pillars in my mind to see if I can pinpoint the problem. Sometimes I realize, "Hey! I haven't worked out in a while," or, "I've been feeling anxious lately and haven't been present," or, "My partner and I really need to address a certain issue before I can desire them again." My hope is that you will use these pillars throughout your sex life to help you take control of your sexuality and start getting the pleasure you desire.

Before you continue on, take a moment to reflect on the five Sex IQ pillars: Embodiment, Health, Collaboration, Self-Knowledge, and Self-Acceptance. Consider where you are in each of these right now and which ones you want to commit to working on. Even if it doesn't seem directly related, all of the advice in this book will help you grow in all of these areas so that you can start having better, smarter sex.

The rest of this book will get into specifics about how to increase your pleasure through masturbation, positions, and different sex acts. As you read, I challenge you to consider these in the context of your Sex IQ. When you do, you'll realize that you're on your way to becoming much smarter about sex.

2

Fight Off the Pleasure Thieves:

The Emotional Blocks Standing Between You and Your Eroticism

Until I reeducated myself about sex and started prioritizing my own pleasure, I led a busy, type A, workaholic life. If I was in a relationship, on Friday nights I'd rush home from work, screech into the driveway, quickly change my clothes, and touch up my makeup for a date with my partner. The whole time, I was stressed-out.

Most likely, I hadn't checked everything off my to-do list, and I had a million "tabs" still open in my brain. Maybe my mom had called me six times and I hadn't called her back yet... Or I had an important meeting the next day that I hadn't finished preparing for... But of course, I wanted to see my boyfriend, so I took my work self, got her dressed up in girlfriend clothes, and got her butt over to see him.

I had been looking forward to our connection and intimacy all week, and more often than not, we headed straight to the bedroom. But once I was there, I couldn't get into it. I didn't feel erotic, sexual, or connected. I didn't feel desire. My body was in bed, but my brain was still in the office. As a result, whatever kind, sexy man I was dating at the time couldn't arouse me no matter how hard he tried. He was no match for my stress, anxiety, and distraction, which quickly spiraled into shame, as my mind went from work to-dos to judgmental thoughts about myself for not being able to relax and enjoy myself.

Just me? Or does any of this sound familiar?

STS: Stress, Trauma, and Shame

It's time to look at the psychological factors that are most likely to undermine your erotic potential—aka the Pleasure Thieves. We each have our own personal cocktail of Pleasure Thieves that are most likely to rear their ugly heads in the bedroom, often based on our upbringing and sexual history. It can be difficult—sometimes even painful—to look back and unearth these suckers, but it's more than worth it. Just becoming aware of your most pervasive thieves and how they manifest in the bedroom can help you steal your pleasure back. I'll also share some tools to fight each of them off, making it infinitely easier to blossom into your most sexual and pleasure-filled self.

The three most common Pleasure Thieves are stress, trauma, and shame. I call them STS for short. Each of these thieves may manifest a little bit differently in each of us. For example, I may respond completely differently than you do to feelings of shame. But I cannot overemphasize how many sexual problems actually have nothing to do with sex itself and have everything to do with these three thieves, instead.

So often, someone asks me for tips on something simple like how to give better oral, and after talking to them for a few minutes it becomes clear that they have internalized deep feelings of shame after being told as a child that genitals are "dirty." That's not a physical problem; it's a psychological one. Like I said earlier, the brain is our biggest sexual organ.

As you read about these thieves, think about which of them resonates with you the most. This is an important way of building Sex IQ pillar #4, Self-Knowledge. Unfortunately, there is usually more than one thief holding us back from having our best possible sex. The good news is that we can work with where you are to combat these thieves and steal back your pleasure.

Pleasure Thief #1: Stress

Stress is the default mode in this culture, but that doesn't mean you have to buy into the idea that being in a constant state of stress is normal. There's a big difference between something being normal and it being *normalized.* It's incredibly common for people to accept stress as a constant part of life or to even pride themselves on it, but this is not healthy and should never have become the norm. And it's quite possibly the number one thing that keeps us from a life of pleasure.

Stress is inevitable, but it can be managed. Again, it starts with awareness. Once you're aware of your stress triggers and how they're impacting your sex life, you will become empowered to start managing your stress. Life as a whole will become more pleasurable, and sexual pleasure will be far more likely to follow. This is the new normal that I want you to move into.

A little reality check, though: you can't eliminate years of stress and anxiety conditioning overnight—or even in several nights. Plus, as I said, a certain amount of stress is normal and even healthy. When something truly scary or threatening happens, you *should* feel stressed. Your body was built to react to these moments with a stress response. It's chronic, never-ending stress that is the real problem and that robs you from pleasure in big and small ways.

To put it simply, stress and pleasure do not mix. We can't have both at the same time because it's not how our bodies were designed. We have two autonomic (involuntary) nervous systems: the sympathetic nervous system, which stimulates the fight, flight, or freeze response (aka the stress response) when activated, and the parasympathetic nervous system, which stimulates the "rest and digest" or "safe and social" response when activated.

Only one of these systems can be activated at a time. They are both essential, biologically and evolutionarily speaking, but only the parasympathetic nervous system allows you to feel pleasure. And stress, whether it's mental, emotional, or physical stress, activates the sympathetic nervous system, instead.

Evolutionarily, this makes complete sense. If you were being chased by a predator, your sympathetic nervous system would activate and all of your resources would go toward helping you run or fight. Your survival is the priority in this case. Why would your body waste energy on activating the sympathetic nervous system in this instance? It wouldn't, and so our bodies are designed so that it can't. In today's world, this translates to feeling a lack of desire when you are in a state of stress, whether or not your survival is actually on the line.

Feeling stressed is antithetical to feeling good. It may seem like your stress is in your head, and that is where it starts, but it affects your entire body. Stress causes an increase in hormones such as cortisol, which triggers the sympathetic nervous system. This causes a decrease in feel-good hormones like serotonin and oxytocin, which virtually kills your sex drive. Chronic stress increases your risk of anxiety and depression, which snuffs out desire, as well.

This happens because when you are stressed, especially long-term, your body is designed to use its resources to help you stay alive, not to have sex. It's when you are calm and relaxed and all is well that your body and brain can prioritize pleasure. This is why your partner may not want to have sex at the end of a long, busy day. It's not you—it's the stress hormones coursing through your partner's body! Why not give them space to practice yoga or something else that relaxes them while you do the dishes, take out the trash, or do something else to help relieve their stress? With your partner now in parasympathetic mode, they will be much more likely to feel erotic desire.

The relationship between stress and pleasure is even more complicated, though. For some people, sex can actually be a powerful stress reliever. And it is true that having an orgasm leads to an increase in those feel-good hormones, serotonin and oxytocin. This is one reason that orgasms are so good for you, which we'll cover in much more depth later on.

If having an orgasm can reduce stress, then why am I saying that stress and pleasure don't mix? It's because having an orgasm to relieve stress is a quick fix. If you don't address the underlying cause of the stress, your hormones will stabilize pretty quickly and then you'll be right back where you started.

More often than not, intense, chronic stress is going to keep you from feeling sexual. When stress is prolonged, the adrenal glands, which produce the stress hormone cortisol, become taxed and cannot function properly. This can lead to a host of other problems and can really do a number on your sex drive.

Listen, I get it. You're a productive person who likes to accomplish a lot. I'm never going to tell you to stop being you. But from one productive hustler to another, I can tell you honestly that I got better at my job when I learned to reduce stress and prioritize pleasure. I've always been a workaholic, and that hasn't really changed. What has changed is my intention in how I schedule my days to prioritize pleasure.

Once I made time for pleasure in real and tangible ways (a morning hike, lunch with friends, frequent masturbation), I experienced a monumental shift. The more pleasure I had, the more productive I was. Plus, I was knocking out tasks with more joy and energy and less resentment and burnout. My pleasure fueled my productivity. Remember, pleasure is productive!

Don't get me wrong—I still have plenty of days when I'm too stressed for pleasure. But now I know what happens when I let stress take over: I no longer want to have sex with my partner and life becomes more filled with anxiety. I feel less pleasure all around.

It's a practice to continue reminding myself that at any moment I have the knowledge and ability to manage my stress and prioritize my pleasure. But when you consciously devote more of your day to pleasurable activities, you start healing those adrenal glands that have been working overtime. In this way, pleasure is not only productive, it's a medicine and a lubricant that can help you create a body that's more ready for sex. This is why I say that to experience your deepest sexual pleasure, you first have to heal your relationship to pleasure in general. Part of this is learning how to manage your stress.

Find Your Pleasure Percent

How much of your day do you currently spend experiencing pleasure? I call the average percentage of your waking hours that you spend doing pleasurable activities your Pleasure Percent. Remember, I'm not just talking about sexual pleasure. I mean anything and everything that feels really good and makes you feel alive.

This may come as a shock, but I recommend shooting for a Pleasure Percent of twenty-five percent of your waking hours, or roughly four hours a day, assuming you sleep for about eight hours at night. (By the way, if you don't get enough sleep, it will increase your stress levels, so aim for eight hours a night.)

I'm sure that right now, twenty-five percent sounds like a lot. I get it. When I first did this exercise, my Pleasure Percent was six. It's taken me years to get it up to twenty-five, and I admit that it often slips back down during extra busy times.

Now, I know how important this is, though, because when you're experiencing pleasure you're in parasympathetic mode, meaning you're relaxed, calm, and present. Spending more time in this state will train your nervous system to get out of sympathetic mode and to stop reacting so strongly to minor stressors. This will lead to better health and a higher quality of life overall, and it will make amazing sex much easier to come by (another pun).

I'm well aware that privilege is a clear and present factor here. Spending a quarter of our waking hours engaging in pleasurable activities is completely inaccessible for far too many of us. We all deserve a life of pleasure and happiness, and it's just wrong that it is only available for some of us.

I keep saying it because it's true: awareness is a great first step. So, let's find out where you're starting from and wherever it is, we can go from there.

By the way, why not make this exercise itself a pleasurable experience? Get out a nice journal, sit down in your favorite chair, and grab a hot cup of tea or coffee or whatever you most enjoy. Pile on a blanket and maybe light a candle. Make this count toward the pleasure percentage of your day! Think about how you can do this when completing other tasks, too.

Step 1:

Take a moment to think about all of the things in your life that give you pleasure of any kind, and then write all of them down. Of course, having sex or masturbating counts, but so does your morning cup of coffee, cuddling with your pet or child or partner, taking a nap or a bath, reading, writing, pursuing a hobby, entertaining friends, things that make you laugh, spending time in nature or with people you love, and even your work—at least, the aspects of your work that you truly enjoy. This can be anything, as long as it is something that brings you genuine pleasure.

Step 2:

Think about the past week. About how much time (in the number of minutes) did you spend doing each activity? Of course, some days might have been busier than others and included very little pleasure time. That's why we're looking at the week as a whole. Look back at your calendar if you need to jog your memory.

For example, if I took a half-hour nap on Saturday, then I would write down thirty as the total number of minutes that I spent napping this week. If I journaled while drinking a nice cup of coffee for ten minutes every morning, I would write down seventy as the total number of minutes I spent on journaling and coffee. You get it. Don't feel pressured to get it perfect here down to the minute. Just make your best guesstimate.

Step 3:

Add up your total number of minutes, regardless of which activity you spent them on. Then divide that total by 960. (This is the number of minutes in sixteen hours, or a waking day.) Now multiply that figure by one hundred. The final number is the percentage of each day that you are currently devoting to pleasure.

If you're scared off by the math, here's an example: if your daily pleasure tally came out to 120 minutes, the equation looks like this: 120 ÷ 960 = .125 x 100 = 12.5 percent.

It's more than likely that your percentage will be

lower than twenty-five—maybe even much lower. That's okay! Start being more intentional about devoting more of your time to pleasure, to the extent that it's possible for you. Even taking small baby steps by adding a few minutes of pleasure a day can really add up. After a few weeks, recalculate your percentage, see how much it has gone up, and keep moving forward from there to a lower stress and more balanced life of pleasure.

Stress Busters

Much has been written about how to manage stress, so I'll keep this part relatively brief, but it is important to review some of the most effective ways to relieve stress and how they directly relate to sex.

Exercise

Moving your body improves your mood, your energy levels, your confidence, and your desire. When someone tells me that their libido is low or they're just not enjoying sex, one of the first things I ask them is whether or not they're getting much exercise. Very often, the answer is no.

Exercise relieves stress by causing your body to release more of those feel-good hormones that soothe the nervous system and less of the stress hormone cortisol. Even better, consistent exercise leads your body to release more endorphins regularly, even when you're not moving your body.

It doesn't matter what kind of exercise you do. Running, yoga, swimming, weight lifting…anything that gets you moving will help relieve stress and boost pleasure. If you can find something that you actually enjoy doing, that's even better.

But wait—there's more. Exercise leads to better sex for another reason that is not directly related to stress, and that is the magic of increased blood flow.

A man in his forties called me recently and asked why his erections were so unpredictable. He was able to get hard sometimes, but not always, and when he did get hard, he couldn't always maintain his erection. By the way, this had nothing to do with his desire to have sex. He wanted to have sex with his partner, and found them incredibly sexy and desirable. He just couldn't make it happen. This is an extremely common problem, so if it happens to you or your partner, know that you are absolutely not alone.

I asked this caller about his overall health—whether or not he was on certain medications, if he smoked, how much he drank, and his eating habits. Overall, he checked off all the boxes and had a clean bill of health. Then I asked him how much he moved in a given day, and—bingo. He sat at a desk all day at his job and hadn't worked out in years.

We talked about how he could start moving every day in small ways, and he agreed to take a daily thirty-minute walk for a month and see how it went. I made him promise to call me back with an update, and when he did, he sounded like a completely different person. He felt more confident and happier overall, and he told me that he'd been inspired to buy some dumbbells and set up a home gym in his garage.

The biggest change in this caller—those pesky erections, of course. He was able to get hard and stay hard much more predictably, all just from thirty minutes of walking per day. This was thanks to increased blood flow. Movement sends blood to the genitals, which in our listener's case, toned the vascularity of his penis.

When you feel desire, blood flow to the genitals is necessary for a physical response—an erection for penis owners or an engorged clitoris for vulva owners. This helps with arousal and ultimately orgasm. Whether you have a penis or a vulva, increased blood flow is a surefire way to improve your orgasms and your overall sex life. Why don't all gyms advertise this?

Breathing

Just like most of us didn't learn much about sex in school, most of us haven't learned about how to breathe, at least not properly. But, as I said earlier, your breath actually has a profound impact on your body, your mind, your nervous system, and your pleasure.

Without proper training, most people breathe shallowly into their lungs. This is also the way we breathe when we are under threat, so it's no surprise that shallow breathing activates the sympathetic nervous system and the stress hormones that go along with it. In other words, shallow breathing equals more stress and less pleasure.

When we breathe deeply, on the other hand, pulling long breaths into and out of our diaphragms, we stimulate the vagus nerve, one of the longest nerves in the human body. Separate from the spinal column, this nerve starts in the brain stem and extends down the neck, to the heart, the lungs, and the digestive system. It regulates and modulates metabolism, some immune functions, and heart rate. But its greatest gift is that it is a de-stressor.

The vagus nerve is basically the off switch for the sympathetic nervous system and the on switch for the parasympathetic nervous system. And the best way to stimulate it is through deep breathing, with exhales that are longer than your inhales.

To stimulate the vagus nerve, I like to do 4-7-8 breathing. To do this, inhale for four seconds, hold your breath for seven seconds, and then exhale slowly for eight seconds. To stimulate and strengthen your vagus nerve, try to practice this breathing technique for fifteen minutes a day. This will make a huge difference in your stress levels and ability to experience pleasure.

Social Interaction

The third way to reduce stress is also the most fun—social interaction. Feeling connected to other humans, whether they are family members, friends, or colleagues, is a natural stress reducer. When we enjoy spending time with people, it increases our levels of oxytocin, and the more oxytocin we have, the more we want to spend time with people. This becomes a positive cycle of more socializing and less stress.

Even casual, quick, positive interactions can boost your mood and shift you into a parasympathetic state. Try to build more of these moments into your day. Compliment a stranger's outfit or give your barista a sincere "Thank you." Maybe even ask how their day is going. You'll be helping them reduce their stress levels, too!

Of course, it matters who you are spending time with. If certain people annoy or trigger you, spending time with them will cause more harm and stress than good. Pay attention to how you feel when you're around different people. The ones that make you feel safe and comfortable and relaxed are the ones you want to intentionally spend more time with.

By the way, another way to stimulate the vagus nerve is by laughing. It's always a good idea to go out of your way to spend more time with those friends and lovers that make you laugh your hardest. Pleasure in the form of laughter is literally healing.

Pleasure Thief #2: Trauma

The word "trauma" can seem loaded and scary, and you might be tempted to skip this section if you think it won't apply to you—but hold on one second. Trauma can simply be defined as an emotional response to a negative event, typically one that makes you feel unsafe. It is not limited to serious incidents like a sexual assault or the death of a loved one. Those are both what I call "big T" traumas, but there are also "little T" traumas, like getting made fun of or a particularly embarrassing moment.

Both "big T" and "little T" traumas, if they're unresolved, can lead to discomfort, fear, anxiety, and apprehension in life and relationships in general and specifically when it comes to sexual pleasure. Even—and sometimes especially—if the trauma happened in the past, it can still be triggering in the present and trip up your ability to fully experience pleasure.

When you're a child, these "little T" traumas add up, because your brain is still being formed. They become a part of us. And because we don't know what to do in those moments, the trauma gets tucked away, metastasizing into learned responses that affect our adult interactions and relationships. You end up having involuntary responses to innocuous events, with no idea why. It's because your sympathetic nervous system reacts automatically when your unresolved traumas are triggered, leaving you stressed and unable to experience pleasure.

Of course, our Pleasure Thieves work together to steal our pleasure any way they can!

To fully experience sexual pleasure, it's essential to figure out what your own history of trauma is and how it's hiding in your body. And by the way—trauma doesn't stop at childhood. Unfortunately, it can happen anytime and often punctuates our childhoods and our adult lives, too.

Of course, I've experienced both big and little traumas of my own. When I was a child, my mother married a man who regularly lost his temper and took it out on my brother and me. He slammed doors, stomped around the house, and berated me for minuscule things, like forgetting to put a pencil back in the drawer. I learned to be incredibly quiet when he was around, ever on guard for his next blowup.

Eventually, I began to hide from my stepfather, running to my room every time I heard him come home from work. I played with my dolls, listened for footsteps outside my door, and in the event that he did come and find me, I turned on my sweetest, most easygoing self. Anything to keep him calm. Anything to ward off the chance that he'd hit me again.

This is "big T" trauma, and my learned response to my stepfather, combined with other types of chaos that I grew up with, eventually became so ingrained that I unconsciously exhibited the same responses with my lovers. Ever the people pleaser, I acted upbeat to a fault with my partners. Instead of seeking my own sexual pleasure with them, I did things to keep them happy. Did they want a blow job? I gave all the blow jobs. Did they want me on top? I climbed on top, moaning and writhing like I'd seen in porn.

By the way, this trauma impacted all areas of my life, not just with sexual partners. To this day, I am a people pleaser and am conflict avoidant in general. It's something that I have to consciously work on. In these moments, the things that help me are reminding myself that I'm responding to past events, taking a few deep breaths, being grateful, redirecting my focus to the present moment, and setting boundaries.

Don't get me wrong. I'm not saying that you shouldn't aim to please your partner. It can be incredibly hot to know that your partner is fully sexually satisfied. But instead of collaborating with my partners to meet *both* of our needs during sex, I completely sacrificed my own pleasure in my efforts to anticipate and prioritize their needs. These men weren't trying to hurt me. I'm sure they wished they knew how to satisfy me. Yet, I was perpetually in service to them.

This is exactly how trauma works: our past experiences create a pattern of hypervigilant and protective responses that dictate our behaviors in the present. In his groundbreaking book, *The Body Keeps the Score: Brain, Mind, and Body in the Healing of Trauma*, Bessel van der Kolk says, "Traumatized people chronically feel unsafe inside their bodies: The past is alive in the form of gnawing interior discomfort. Their bodies are constantly bombarded by visceral warning signs."

In its external form, we each wear our own trauma differently, from person to person. Trauma can lead to post-traumatic stress disorder, anxiety, depression, shame, self-loathing, substance abuse, disordered eating, toxic relationships, fear of sex, fear of people, isolation, mistrust of the legal and medical professions, and so on. What do all of these things have in common? They are your body's way of trying to keep you safe when it believes you are constantly in danger.

So, how can we fully enjoy pleasure when our bodies are trying a little *too* hard to protect us? The first step, as always, is awareness. As Van der Kolk says, "Physical self-awareness is the first step in releasing the tyranny of the past."

Trauma can have a profound impact on your sex life because it prevents you from being open and vulnerable. To have a fulfilling sex life, you have to be able to drop your defenses and be vulnerable. If you are constantly on high alert, even when you're with someone you love, you won't be able to have the sex life you deserve and desire.

Start paying attention to the ways your body responds to different experiences. When you feel that you've overreacted to something, ask yourself why. Did it remind you of something from the past? Even if the situation wasn't exactly the same, there may have been something about it that your body picked up on as familiar.

For example, when I was in my twenties, I never would have dreamed that rough touch could be sexy. Are you kidding me? I still carried old associations of my stepfather, so when a partner reared back to give me a playful spank, I tensed up. It wasn't hot; it was scary.

After taking time to learn about my trauma, understand its sources, and make conscious decisions to create new connections, pleasure became my ally. Many people think that you have to completely heal your trauma in order to experience your full capacity for pleasure. But I have found that it's actually the other way around: experiencing pleasure and focusing my awareness on that pleasure has helped me counterbalance the emotional effects of trauma.

When we familiarize our body with safety and delight, we give our nervous system the medicine it needs. Little by little, we're dosing ourselves with joy, reminding our body that we are safe, and that we are living in a different story and reality now.

Another important step for me was therapy. Next to lube, this is probably the number one thing I recommend. For me, working with a counselor who specializes in EMDR (eye movement desensitization and reprocessing) was crucial to understanding and releasing the severity of my trauma. EMDR allows us to reprocess memories that were stored in the brain in ways that cause distress. It rewires your brain to react differently to a similar or triggering event in the future.

Movement can also help. It will reduce your stress, and by mindfully engaging in physical activities, you can rewire your brain's associations with specific sensations of pleasure instead of danger. I'm also a fan of exposure therapy, which involves reapproaching a frightening situation in the safety of a therapeutic setting. This helps your brain refile it from the horror folder to the neutral folder. It's all about putting mind and body back in alignment.

After years of therapy and allowing myself to invite pleasure into my life, I now live in a body that's freer and more trusting, especially during sex. This can be your future, too.

Pleasure Thief #3: Shame

"Shame" is one of those words that we've all heard, but when it comes to pleasure, it's helpful to know precisely what we're talking about. A lot of people use the words "shame" and "guilt" interchangeably, but in truth, they're attached to two different sets of beliefs. As Brené Brown says, guilt is a feeling of "I did something bad," while shame goes deeper. It is a feeling of "I *am* bad."

To apply this to sex, try switching out the word "bad" for another negative descriptor. Maybe it's "I am unattractive," or "I'm bad at sex," or "I'm morally dirty." Because shame is wrapped up in identity, these descriptors have a sense of permanence to them, manifesting in narratives that we create about ourselves. These are things like "I'm ugly, and no one would want to have sex with me," or "There must be something wrong with me if this turns me on."

I can't begin to tell you the number of people who reach out to me for reassurance that they aren't sexual deviants just because they watch a lot of porn or want to try anal sex. And time after time, the question they're really asking is "Is there something wrong with me? Am I normal?" This is a question that is completely wrapped in shame—shame that keeps them from exploring their sexuality and fully experiencing pleasure.

To root out any shame that may be stealing your pleasure, we need to identify the type you may be experiencing. I have identified four shame patterns around sex and pleasure that trigger a common set of fears:

- Rejection
- Exposure
- Self-Blame
- Internalized Judgment

If you, like me, have experienced all four of these types of shame at some point, I promise you aren't broken. Shame thrives in secrecy, but when we shine a light on it, we neutralize its power and stop it from stealing our pleasure.

Rejection Shame

Those of us with rejection shame fear that deep down, we are fundamentally unlovable. It follows that it would be easy for our partners to leave us, so we typically try to preempt this by doing everything we can to make them stay. This often manifests in people pleasing and sacrificing our own pleasure for theirs instead of collaborating mutually.

In practical terms, here's what rejection shame looks like in the bedroom: faking orgasms, performing sex acts you don't really want to do just because your partner wants to, and generally acting out of fear of being turned away, not from a place of desire.

The origin of this kind of shame can come from having a critical or absent parent as a child. It can stem from experience with critical partners, too. If someone once put you down during sex, it could cause you to forever monitor yourself for perceived flaws.

I remember a caller whose ex-boyfriend tried to pressure her into having anal sex. He called her a prude for not wanting to try it. Worse, he compared her unfavorably to one of his past partners, saying, "I wish you were a little more sexually open, like she was."

That one phrase—"I wish you were a little more sexually open"—stayed in her head for years, prompting her to do all kinds of sex acts that she didn't really want or enjoy. She didn't want to be rejected again and thought that acting more sexually liberated would make her more lovable.

Once she realized that she was acting on her fear of being rejected, she was able to focus on what she really wanted sexually instead of doing what she thought her partners wanted of her. Then she shared this information with her future partners and got ahead of it by telling them that she sometimes worried about not being open sexually and that it was important to her to be a with a partner who was open to talk about sex.

No matter what anyone has said or how they have treated

you, you are lovable and worthy of love and pleasure. You do not have to change anything about yourself in order to be loved. Period, end of story.

Exposure Shame

This is the fear of being "found out," or someone discovering something about you that is horrible and "wrong." Exposure shame usually stems from a humiliating experience: getting caught masturbating and the other person reacting with shock and horror, or getting caught up in a sexual moment, only to have your raw vulnerability pierced by a withering comment.

Many vulva owners refuse to receive oral sex because, once upon a time, someone told them they smelled bad, or they heard that vaginas were unsanitary and unattractive. Now this is the only thing they can think about each and every time a partner starts moving down their body, teasing their underwear away. What could be so hot and pleasurable is instead a major source of anxiety. Instead of thinking, "Damn, this feels amazing," they are thinking, "It's only moments before they realize I smell/look/taste awful!"

Left unprocessed, this type of shame limits your pleasure potential because it leaves you trapped by a secret that you feel you have to keep. The irony is that many of these secret sources of shame are actually completely normal, but most people don't realize that because they never talk about sex! Well, until now.

For example, I get calls all the time from listeners who feel so much shame about never orgasming from penetrative sex (normal), the fact that their genitals smell a little different from one day to the next (normal), or the fact that sometimes they prefer masturbating to having sex with their partner (normal).

What are you hiding? It's probably become so much bigger in your mind than it is in reality. Later in the book, we'll talk about how to communicate with our partners about every aspect of sex. Airing out these secrets will likely help the shame dissipate. You'll also find that as you evolve in all of your Sex IQ pillars and accept yourself more, you will be less afraid of others learning the truth about you. The more you accept yourself, the more you'll trust that others will help you, too.

Self-Blame Shame

Those of us with self-blame shame take on responsibility for other people's thoughts, feelings, actions, and even sexual pleasure. A classic (and somewhat clichéd) self-blame shame origin story is a child listening to their parents fight at dinner and thinking, "This started because I spilled my juice. It's my fault. If I never spill anything again, they won't argue anymore." The self-blaming child takes on an undue amount of responsibility for their parents' happiness, assuming that they are the primary reason behind their parents' stress. Later if that child's parents got divorced, the child might sadly blame themselves for that, too.

At its core, self-blame shame is a way that we attempt to take back some control in an out-of-control situation. On some level, we figure that if we're the problem, at least there's a way to fix it.

As adults, self-blame shame manifests as low self-esteem, self-sabotage, codependent relationships, and the belief that when bad things happen to us, we deserve it. It can also look like an extreme fear of abandonment (rejection shame), locking people into unsatisfying or unhealthy relationships because they believe it's the best they deserve. They confuse healthy humility with self-sabotage, believing that they're somehow responsible for people treating them badly.

In the bedroom, self-blame shame can manifest as feeling bad about ourselves if our partner can't maintain an erection or have an orgasm or even if they're not in the mood. To someone with self-blame shame, all of these examples could be signs that they're not attractive enough or are a bad lover. Outside of the bedroom, they might take responsibility for their partner's bad mood, feeling the need to fix everything.

I say it all the time because it's true: you are responsible for your own pleasure. That means that your partner is responsible for their own pleasure, too! Work together, but at the end of the day, you can't control anyone but yourself, and you're not responsible for anyone else's behavior, emotions, or orgasms.

Internalized Judgment Shame

When it comes to sex, internalized judgment is one of the most common flavors of shame I see. Belonging is a primal need, and to belong, we often feel that we need to be "normal," whatever the hell that means. And it's so easy to fall into the habit of trying to contort ourselves into what we think is normal, while feeling shame when we don't fit neatly into that box.

A big source of internalized judgment shame that keeps us from the pleasure we deserve is body insecurity. For decades, we've been on the receiving end of messaging that tells us only certain types of people deserve sexual pleasure. Most mainstream porn and sexy scenes in other media feature young, thin, and mostly white bodies. Many of us assume that if we don't look like those people, then we must not deserve pleasure and we should be ashamed of the way we look.

But here's the truth: that is a lie. We all deserve pleasure no matter how old we are or what we look like. All of us. It is our birthright as human beings.

I can't even begin to tell you how many penis owners I speak to who have internalized judgment shame about their penis size or shape. They think that their partners won't want to have sex with them if their penis is a little crooked or isn't ten inches long like the ones they see in porn. Penis owners spend so much time worrying about their penis size that it keeps them from experiencing pleasure.

First of all, I promise that no one cares about your penis as much as you do! The average penis size is about five and a half inches, nothing like what is depicted in most porn. And, most important, penis size is not an indicator of being a great lover. The vast majority of vulva owners experience more pleasure and orgasms from the mouth, hands, or toys than from a penis. So, stop worrying about your penis, and start fully enjoying your pleasure.

Getting rid of internalized judgment shame begins with questioning our ideas of normal when it comes to sex. Our goal isn't just to celebrate our individuality. It's to acknowledge that there is no normal. Again, for the people in the cheap seats—there is no normal. There are some things that are common. There are others that are normalized. But there is no one right way to look or to be in order to have sex or to experience pleasure.

Reframing Shame

The very language that we use around shame is problematic. Take the word "shameless," for example. It means being amoral, brazen, or selfish. If you are shameless, we're told, you are a terrible person. Does that mean that if you are full of shame, you are a good person? Goodness should not be synonymous with having shame, but our language and culture tells us that it is.

To reframe and ultimately get rid of this nasty Pleasure Thief, try to see it as a download that was installed in you by someone else. Look into your past and think about where your shame came from. How did it first get into your hard drive? Who installed it? Many of us grew up in houses in which sex was seen as shameful, and our society reinforces shame in so much of the content we see about sex in movies, on TV, and on social media.

Next, start to notice how shame is affecting you. What happens in your mind and body that allows this thief to steal your pleasure? Ask yourself, "What was I thinking and doing right before I felt it?" Were you talking to your mother? Were you thinking about something an ex said in the past? Were you hungry? Angry? Lonely? Tired? With someone? Comparing yourself to someone else? Feeling judged or criticized? Waiting for someone to call, email, or text you back? Connect the dots from the present trigger to the past when the wound first opened.

Practically speaking, you can start to shift the feelings of shame by using movement and breath. Do a few push-ups, go for a walk in the fresh air, or take some deep breaths to reset. Social interaction can help, too. By sharing your feelings of shame with a trusted friend, partner, or therapist, you'll feel connected, less alone, and not broken.

Another clear path out of shame is to focus on what actually feels good. Explore your body. People who have been shut down to sexual pleasure are often unable to feel good about *anything.* Take baby steps toward accepting pleasure. You won't go from shame-filled to shame-free overnight. But with practice, you'll fight off feelings of shame and reclaim the life of pleasure that you deserve.

Exercise: Flip the Script

Every type of shame that we've covered stems from a narrative that belongs to someone else, but that we have taken on as our truth. No more. Now we get to write our own stories around sex and pleasure, and here's your chance to start that process.

When I do call-in shows and take ten callers at random, consistently half of them are people from religious backgrounds who were raised to believe that they don't deserve pleasure. For them, masturbating poses a moral conflict. Every time they want to feel sexual pleasure, they feel in their bones like they're wronging their parents, priest, and the church, even though they know deep down that it's not true.

When I ask them how it feels, they say that they start to feel tension in their chest. That shame is embodied.

It's buried inside of them. And your shame is, too. You can tap into that feeling and identify it.

When you start to feel ashamed of something, ask yourself, "What am I feeling?" Write it down. Next, ask yourself, "What narrative goes with that feeling?" If you were told that whatever you're doing is sinful, write that down. For example, "I feel like oral sex is sinful."

This is the mental sexual script that was written for you by someone else that got stuck in your mind. It does not have to be your truth. Flip the script by writing the opposite with an "and" intention. For example, "I felt like oral sex is virtuous, *and* I'm prioritizing pleasure, joy, and self-care because they are important to me."

If you feel ashamed of yourself for making time for pleasure, write down, "I don't deserve pleasure and joy."

Then, write the opposite plus an "and" statement: "I deserve pleasure, *and* that means taking daily walks, spending time with friends, and masturbating a few times a week."

Trying on these new stories might feel strange at first, or even forced. The trick here is familiarity. Those old stories feel comfortable and familiar and therefore safe. Now you're exposing them for what they are—someone else's belief system—and replacing them with your actual, authentic truth. In time, these new stories will start to feel familiar and *right* to your mind and body. No longer carrying other people's hang-ups, your body will start to sink into a state of rest and relaxation—exactly what you need to start feeling desire again and take your pleasure back.

Ultimately, the Pleasure Thieves take away our pleasure by taking us out of the moment. As pleasure is presence, any thoughts that pop up about our wiggly bellies, our cellulite, a sink full of dirty dishes, or a painful sexual encounter will distract us from fully experiencing and enjoying sex. Some of these are easier to get over than others. It may take some time. Be patient with yourself—remember, self-judgment is a Pleasure Thief—and work on accepting where you are right now. This will help you grow your self-acceptance and fight off these Pleasure Thieves for good.

3

You Do You:

How (and Why) to Make Your Solo Sex Magical

It will probably come as no surprise to hear that when I was growing up, no one talked to me about masturbating. I didn't even really know it was a thing, especially not for vulva owners. The only images I saw of masturbation were in comedic teen movies like *Porky's* and *Fast Times at Ridgemont High*, and those movies just showed awkward penis owners going into a bathroom, sitting on the toilet, and making funny faces. I barely had any idea what was happening, but I intuited that it probably had something to do with sex and that it was definitely embarrassing, maybe even shameful.

I eventually figured out what all those funny faces were about, but by the time I was in college, I still hadn't bothered to try it for myself. At around that time, some of my friends finally started opening up and talking about masturbation. Of course, no one had talked to them about masturbating, either, and they shared stories about how they had accidentally stumbled onto their first orgasms—often while riding a bike, grinding against a pillow, or even using an electric toothbrush.

Honestly, I was confused. I'd ridden bikes. I had pillows and toothbrushes. But I hadn't developed a deep, personal relationship with any of these objects. When one of my friends mentioned bathtub jets, I finally decided to try it for myself. We had a tub with jets at home, so when I was at home for my next break, I decided to give it a whirl.

After a few tries, I was finally able to position myself so the jets hit me in the right spot. I was slowly starting to relax into the sensations I was feeling when my mom came into the bathroom without knocking and found me straddling the tub. A complete masturbation novice, I had forgotten to lock the door.

My mom looked horrified, I was mortified, and we never spoke of it again.

It would take me several more years before I started masturbating successfully and regularly, this time with the help of a vibrator instead of the bathtub. I still wasn't having orgasms with my partners. I enjoyed the connection during sex, and receiving oral sex felt good, but I still wasn't able to orgasm. I continued the bad habit of faking it, and that first orgasm I had using a vibrator was quite the eye-opener.

After all this time, I finally started to understand what all the fuss was about. All along, I'd had the power and ability to feel that explosive, magical, fully satisfying release. Why hadn't anyone told me?

Until then, I had been living with the misconception that penis owners should know how to please a vulva. I assumed that either they were born with this knowledge, or they learned it during a secret lesson in middle school while vulva owners were separated to learn about their periods. I truly had no idea that most penis owners are just as clueless about how to please a vulva as many vulva owners are themselves. They didn't have some secret owner's manual. It was a huge relief to learn that we all have insecurities in the bedroom and that my partners didn't know any more about my body than I did. We were in this together.

Let this be your encouragement to create and write your body's owner's manual. Use the notes app in your phone and track the types of touch, positions, and situations that bring you pleasure. Then you can educate your partners about how you like to be pleased. By the way, this goes for penis owners, too.

When I did this, I discovered so many different erogenous zones. I was able to have internal orgasms, more nipple pleasure, and direct my partner where to place his finger to guarantee a blended orgasm. Once I started paying attention and sharing this information with partners, they were always grateful for the knowledge. I could visibly see them release years of pressure and shame they had placed on themselves to get it right.

Since then, masturbation has been one of my favorite topics and activities. My goal with all of my work is to liberate the conversation about sex, and talking about masturbation is a huge and essential part of that.

Solo Sex Is Self-Care

Developing a masturbation practice, or as I call it, having solo sex, is step one on your journey toward reaching your pleasure potential. I'm literally begging you not to skip this step because it's one of the most important ones that infiltrates every pillar of your Sex IQ. Every one of us has the ability to experience profound pleasure, and our bodies contain all of the information we need to discover what makes us feel good. We owe it to ourselves (and to our partners) to figure it out for ourselves and by ourselves. Even if you're already having great sex, but you're not currently having regular solo sex, I promise you that adding in this step will make the rest of your explorations that much more satisfying.

If you're hesitant about masturbation, this is a great time to check which Pleasure Thief is keeping you from having a healthy solo sex practice. Are you feeling shame about exploring your body, or does it relate to trauma? I encourage you to work through those blocks because getting to know your own body and what makes it sing is probably the most fun, exciting work that a human can do. It will help you discover what brings you to orgasm and allow you to gain so much more self-knowledge in general.

Through solo sex, you'll learn what turns you on, what type of physical sensations you like, what parts of your body are the most sensitive, what sorts of fantasies you'd like to explore further, and so much more. I'll go so far as to say that the majority of sexual breakthroughs that you'll have throughout your life will be during solo and not partnered sex.

But hang on, because it gets even better! Solo sex is a powerful—and even necessary—form of self-care. I'm not talking about the commercialized type of self-care that involves buying things or grooming yourself to fit into a fabricated standard of beauty. I'm talking about the kind of self-care that is good for your mind, body, and soul.

Part of the reason that masturbation is such a powerful form of self-care is that it liberates us from the performative aspects of partnered sex. I'm in no way knocking sex with a partner, but let's be honest—it can come with a lot of pressure. We want to please our partners and make sure they know we're having a good time. Plus, even the most confident among us have some level of self-consciousness around our bodies—how they look and smell and taste, the strange and embarrassing sounds they might make, and the fluids that are released during sex. It's a lot, and it can all seriously distract us from our own pleasure.

But solo sex is an opportunity to indulge in pleasure strictly for pleasure's sake with no one and nothing to distract you and no one else to please but yourself. I can't think of anything more body-and-soul nourishing than that. I have also seen so many times how masturbation can help us heal. The more intimate self-knowledge you gather and the more you experience pleasure, the further you will step into being the empowered, incredible, pleasure-loving person that you were born to be.

Solo sex is also self-care because it is good for your health. Every time you have solo sex, your body releases the hormones that make you feel happy, energized, and motivated like serotonin, oxytocin, dopamine, and endorphins. This means that solo sex decreases stress, our number one Pleasure Thief, opening us up to more and more pleasure.

Masturbation also strengthens Sex IQ pillar #5, Self-Acceptance. The more one-on-one time you have with your genitals, the deeper connection you'll build with these parts of you that can give you so much pleasure. There will be little room for self-criticism when you're mindfully connected.

Solo sex also boosts our moods and helps ease symptoms of anxiety and depression, soothes menstrual cramps and helps regulate menstrual cycles for vulva owners, increases our self-esteem, helps us get better sleep, and even boosts our immune systems! Remember that next cold and flu season.

Clearly, Mother Nature wants us to engage in solo sex. So, why aren't more of us doing it? Well, many of us were raised to believe that solo sex is dirty or wrong or morally shameful. We've also been inundated with myths and straight-up lies about why solo sex is bad for us and will harm our sex lives, even though the opposite is true.

Let's clear this up once and for all. Penis owners, you are not "wasting your seed" by masturbating. Sperm is regenerative. You are not going to run out of it. You're also not going to go blind or grow hair on your palms from masturbating, in case you didn't already know that. And vulva owners, you are not going to get addicted to your vibrator or become numb to your partner's touch if you use one. Solo sex also isn't just for "sad," "desperate," "lonely" singles. Solo sex is for all of us to learn, explore, play, and indulge.

Yes, please! Sign me up. Plus, your present and/or future relationships will be stronger if you engage in solo sex. Pleasure begets pleasure, and sex begets sex. By keeping your pilot light lit, you'll find yourself simmering away, ready and excited for more sex with your partner.

Heads-up—this also means that it's just as important and healthy for your partner to engage in solo sex, too. For many of us, this idea triggers fears of inadequacy. We worry that if our partner masturbates, it means that we're not enough for them. This may be hard to hear, but the truth is that your partner's solo sex has nothing to do with you—just like yours has nothing to do with them.

I get it, though. When I was still in my twenties, I was having the best sex of my life with my partner. I was more satisfied in that relationship than I'd ever been. And then, one day, I found his porn collection.

It turned out that my boyfriend's favorite porn star was a blonde woman with huge breasts, while I'm a brunette with breasts that are on the smaller size. I'm not proud of it, but I freaked out, and immediately felt insecure, betrayed, and incredibly jealous—all because I assumed that if he masturbated while watching or thinking about this other woman, it meant that he'd rather be having sex with her or with someone who looked like her than with me. I wasn't enough for him.

It took me a long time to unlearn assumptions like these, and I totally understand why many of us still hold on to them. We feel threatened if we're not the only ones who drive our partners wild. But that's not how life works. We simply don't get to control anyone else's thoughts or actions or fantasies or turn-ons. We don't get to control anyone else's pleasure, and no one else gets to control ours.

No matter how hot and sexy you are and how amazing your sex life with your partner is, they are going to find other people attractive because they are human—and so are you! When we develop our own rich fantasy life, it adds color and dimension to our erotic imaginations.

Anything that your partner watches or thinks about while masturbating is not a replacement for you. Instead, think of it as an add-on or an enhancement.

Pleasure, like love, is an infinite resource. The well does not run dry.

Your Pleasure Parts

There are so many exciting, sensitive parts of your body for you to explore during solo sex. Many of us never learned about them and don't know what many of them even are. We only know the basics: penis and vagina, which isn't even exactly right! Here is a refresher on all of the many fascinating parts of your genitals that can bring you tremendous pleasure.

For Vulva Owners:

Vulva: The entire external genital area. This includes the mons pubis, labia minora, labia majora, and the clitoris.

Mons pubis: The rounded mass of fatty tissue lying over the joint of the pubic bone—the part where pubic hair grows. It's loaded with nerve endings.

Clitoral hood: The skin that covers the clitoris and is similar to penile foreskin. It retracts when aroused.

Clitoris: Swells when aroused, contains thousands of nerve endings, and connects to legs called crura that reach deeply inside the body.

Labia majora: The palace gates: the large, hairy, fleshy outer lips of the vulva. There are a lot of nerve endings here, so these can feel amazing when aroused.

Labia minora: The symmetrical smaller inner lips that surround the vaginal opening and swell during sexual stimulation. These are also sensitive because of nerve endings and are a source of pleasure.

Vagina: The muscular tube through which menstrual blood and babies pass. The outer third is the most sensitive because the clitoral legs are in that region.

G-spot: An internal region located about two inches inside of the vagina, perched on the front vaginal wall, known to provide pleasure and orgasms. The G-spot was named after German gynecologist Ernst Gräfenberg, who first discovered it, although I prefer to call it the "G-area," because it's really more of an area than a spot.

A-spot: The anterior fornix erogenous zone or AFE zone or A-spot is located between the front vaginal wall and the cervix, about four to five inches inside the vagina. Stimulating the A-spot can lead to lubrication and even orgasm.

U-spot: Positioned at the opening of the vagina, directly above and to either side of the urethral opening, the U-spot is very sensitive to light touch.

Skene's glands: Located on either side of the urethra, these glands secrete mucus-containing fluids when stimulated. They help with vaginal lubrication and are responsible for the fluids that come out during female ejaculation. (Yes, this is a thing!)

Pudendal nerve: The major nerve in the pelvic region that is responsible for orgasm, running through the pelvic floor muscles and sending motor and sensation info to and from the genitals.

Bartholin's glands: Glands located on each side of the vaginal opening, secreting fluid that helps lubricate the vagina.

Vestibule: The area of flesh surrounding the opening of the vagina.

Anus: The end point of the digestive system, containing tons of pleasurable nerve endings.

Perineum: The area between the anus and the vaginal opening, which is typically very sensitive.

P-spot: The posterior fornix is located near the cervix on the posterior wall. It is most easily accessed with fingers, a penis, or toy in a rear entry position.

K-spot: Often referred to as the "kundalini" spot, this area is located where the vagina ends and the cervix begins. This location makes the K-spot difficult to access.

For Penis owners:
Penis: The whole unit: the shaft, head, and frenulum. The penis head is rich with nerve endings.

Frenulum: The notch on the underside of the penis where the shaft meets the head. This is the most sensitive area of a circumcised penis.

Foreskin: Sheath covering the head that retracts when

the penis is erect. This is the most sensitive area of an uncircumcised penis.

Scrotum and testes: The ball sac and balls inside of it. Some people like a light touch here, some like intense touch, and some like no touch at all because it's too sensitive.

Prostate: A walnut-shaped gland located two inches inside of the rectum, toward the belly button. For many penis owners, the prostate brings immense pleasure when stimulated.

Shaft: The long part of the penis that connects the head to the lower belly.

Corpora cavernosa and corpus spongiosum: Columns of spongy tissue inside the shaft that fill with blood and trap it in order to make an erection.

Corona: The rounded border at the base of the penis.

Perineum: The area between the anus and the scrotum, which is typically very sensitive.

Anus: The end point of the digestive system, containing tons of pleasurable nerve endings.

For further reference, please see the illustrations of the vulva and penis anatomy on pages 150 and 153.

Mindful Masturbation

Many of us who masturbate regularly already know how to "rub one out" quickly. It's very routine. We grab our favorite toy or turn on our favorite porn and touch ourself exactly how we know will make us orgasm. There's nothing wrong with this! I refer to this type of solo sex as maintenance masturbation. When you don't have a lot of time or just need a quick release, a little round of maintenance masturbation can really hit the spot (in more ways than one).

However, as you begin to further explore your body and your pleasure, I encourage you to try something a little different, which I call mindful masturbation.

Mindfulness is all about being present and taking in all sensory input in the moment. To practice being more mindful, simply start tuning in to your senses. As you're reading these words, what sensations can you feel? Is there something you can smell? Any sounds that you hear?

As I said earlier, pleasure is presence because you must be present when you are experiencing the heights of sexual pleasure. Being present during your entire solo sex session will therefore make it more pleasurable. Who doesn't want that?

Mindful masturbation is not about squeezing an orgasm into your day. It's about taking the time to explore your sensuality. Before you get started, set the mood as if you were having a date come over. Clear the clutter, which can be stressful and distracting, light a candle, turn on some music, and lie down on some nice, soft sheets.

Instead of going right for the genitals, focus on a few other pleasure zones first. You're seducing yourself here, so go nice and slow like the attentive lover that you are. Take some time to caress your neck and see what kind of pressure feels good—maybe a light stroke or a gentle squeeze. How does it feel with one hand versus both? Maybe move on to your nipples and experiment there, too, with soft touches, squeezes, strokes, and even some light tugs.

Moving your hands down your body from your waist to your thighs, see how it feels to touch softly and then apply slightly more pressure as you explore your belly, hips, and inner thighs. Play with all kinds of touch—tickles, light scratches, or a more forceful squeeze.

As you dive into these explorations, make a mental note to label your feelings in your owner's manual. Which touch brought up excitement? Joy? Anticipation? What types of touch brought up feelings of discomfort? What parts of your body felt numb? Which were the most sensitive? There are no right or wrong answers here at all. You're simply mapping your body and getting more attuned to its preferences.

If any intrusive thoughts like "This is silly" or "This feels wrong" or "I hate my body" arise (and, let's be real, they probably will) acknowledge them and then return to your breath. Taking a few deep breaths is a great way to restart everything. Breathe, breathe, breathe, and then go back to the moment—"Okay, where was I? I'm tracing my fingers along my inner thigh, which makes me slightly shiver..." Practice tensing and relaxing your pelvic floor muscles to continually bring your connection back to your genitals.

About this time, you also might start to feel impatient and wonder if you're getting there. It was a game changer when I realized that part of the practice is bringing yourself back to the present moment—even if you have to do it twenty times, and you probably will. Remember, there is no "there" there. You are simply present in the moment, exploring your body's sensations. There is no goal. Your pleasure is its own reward.

Mindful Masturbation for Vulvas

If you've followed the prep steps above, you've now dropped into an ideal headspace for genital exploration: you're present, you're embodied, and you're encouraging blood flow to all the right places.

I recommend you start with a practice called Vulva Cupping to ground yourself before you get started. Warm up by using the palm of your hands to cup your vulva. You can do this either over your panties or under. Feel free to hold your hand there as long as you'd like. Then gently rock your hips back and forth to create stimulation without moving your hands away.

This practice helps me reset, calms anxiety, and helps me connect to my body. For many vulva owners who feel very disconnected from their bodies, this might be a tool to connect for the first time! It's a powerful practice, and eventually you can teach a partner how to do it as part of a foreplay or simply as a grounding ritual.

When you're ready to move on, use your fingers or a toy or both to start to touch the outer labia, which can also stimulate internal clitoral nerves. They are made of highly sensitive erectile tissue, so explore here with different types of touches, including rubs, light tugs, and maybe even a tiny pinch.

Go exceptionally slow to give your nerve endings time to register what's happening. Some of us have more nerve endings here than others, so for some it might feel too sensitive while for others it might feel perfect, and for still others it might feel numb. Any and all of these are completely normal.

Now find the clitoris. The clitoris is the only body part that exists exclusively for pleasure. Some of its nerve endings sit closer to the top of the skin, while thousands more reach deeper inside connecting to your larger clitoral network. Using a finger, experiment with touch here, noticing what feels good. Try light tapping, rubbing, small circles, harder pressure, and softer pressure.

You can also mentally divide your clitoris into quadrants, placing your finger on each quadrant one at a time until sensations arise. Some people find the top left quadrant is the most sensitive part of their clitoris. For others, it's the bottom right. Talk about valuable information! It's helpful to use a mirror to follow along. As you explore, notice if there is a quadrant that's more responsive to your touch than the others.

As you become more aroused, your genitals will become engorged with blood, which will make it easier for you to find your

G-spot. Again, go very, very slowly here, listening to your body to feel precisely what happens when you stimulate the vaginal canal. Locate the front wall of the vagina, and using a "come here" motion with your index finger, place pressure one to two inches up. You're feeling for a slightly raised, bumpy patch of skin. That's your G-spot, and right above it is the A-spot, or anterior fornix. You can also check out the U-spot, positioned at the opening of the vagina, directly above and to either side of the urethral opening.

If you've never heard of the A-spot or the U-spot, you're far from alone. New discoveries about sexual anatomy are being made all the time, especially when it comes to vulvas, which historically have not been a highly funded area of research.

Now you're getting a good idea of what feels good and where. Keep going. If you finish your mindful masturbation session with an orgasm, good for you, but that is not a requirement or a mark of your success. I'll keep saying it until you embody that truth. If you spent time with yourself being present and embodied, consider it a job well done.

Mindful Masturbation for Penises

Most penis owners don't need to be told or reminded to masturbate. Generally speaking, if you have a penis, chances are that you've already explored it. The goal here, then, is to slow down, discover ways to orgasm without using porn (if that's your go-to), and to feel more in control of your orgasm.

Start by placing your fingers around the shaft of your penis, using your nondominant hand. Many penis owners get so used to their own grip and rhythm that they have a hard time orgasming during partnered sex. So, when masturbating mindfully, a great way to break this pattern is to switch up your grip. Try a different rhythm, too. If you always go up and down, try moving diagonally. Stroke yourself from side to side or twist your hand around.

Stay curious and go slow. You might make a big discovery about what you like—or what you don't. Both types of information are equally valuable.

Make sure to take some time to focus on the head of the penis. Just like with the clitoris, you can divide the head into quadrants and linger on each quadrant as you apply pressure, trying to pinpoint which one feels the most sensitive. Think about using your free hand to stimulate your frenulum and your testes. These are highly underrated erogenous zones.

Experiment with different qualities of touch on your frenulum. Now very gently cup your testes in your hand and squeeze. Does it feel great or do you want more pressure? Is it too sensitive to any touch at all? Any and all answers are correct! Simply pay attention as you learn about your body and all of the ways it likes to receive pleasure.

How Much Is Too Much?

Despite being a huge fan of solo sex, I do want to add a quick word of warning that it is possible for this to become a compulsive behavior, along with watching porn. I don't want the fear of becoming too reliant to keep you from experiencing the full erotic pleasures of solo sex, so simply keep an eye out for these warning signs. Frequent masturbation is only a problem if you can no longer get turned on by your partner, you find yourself making excuses to get out of having sex with them so that you can go it alone (although this might be more of a relationship problem than a masturbation problem), and/or you're missing work or other important events so you can stay home and stimulate yourself.

Likewise, watching porn is not bad and it's certainly nothing to be ashamed of, but it can become a problem if you are skipping or ducking out of gatherings so you can watch more of it, if you feel compelled to watch porn in public places like the subway or in line at the grocery store, you can't become aroused or have an orgasm unless you're looking at porn, or you can only get an erection if porn is on in the background.

Another warning sign is escalation—aka jumping on the hedonic treadmill. For example, you used to be satisfied with videos of threesomes, but that isn't enough for you anymore, so you find yourself moving on to porn depicting gang bangs. If you ever feel unsettled by the content of what you're watching, that's a clear indication that you've crossed a line.

People who are addicted to porn or to excessive masturbation (or to any substance) often feel powerless and worthless, which is also shame inducing. The first step, as always, is admitting that you have a problem and that you feel powerless over your decisions. Then you can pursue effective treatments like cognitive behavioral therapy, acceptance and commitment therapy, psychotherapy, twelve-step programs, and/or couples counseling.

If you're not exhibiting any of these warning signs, then you get to decide for yourself how often it feels right for you to masturbate. Two to three solo sex sessions a week is a reasonable, healthy benchmark for any of us, but if you can masturbate every day without consequences—e.g., you're not hurting yourself, you're still able to get turned on by a partner, and you're not taking time away from other important areas of your life—who am I to stop you?

Self-Pleasure Enhancers

You don't need a lot of bells and whistles to fully enjoy mindful masturbation, but, let's be honest, a few vibrating bells and sexy whistles never hurt anyone. Here are some ideas to help take your solo sessions to the next level, and for additional self-pleasure enhancing references, scan the QR code in the references section at the end of the book.

Fantasy

Many of us like the mental stimulation of imagining an exciting sexual scene while we're masturbating, while others prefer visual stimulation (pictures or porn). If you already know what kinds of fantasies you like, good for you. If you haven't tried fantasizing or aren't sure what sorts of fantasies even turn you on, you're not alone. I've never been a natural at conjuring up sexual fantasies myself.

To get started, simply allow your mind go where it wants to go while you're touching yourself. Maybe you'll conjure a scene from a particularly hot session with a present or past partner. Or maybe your mind will imagine something novel that you're curious about—group sex, threesomes, two vulva owners together, or two penis owners together. The options are endless!

Don't judge or edit yourself here or let that Pleasure Thief shame take this fun experience away from you. The thoughts that pop into your head are not messages from your subconscious instructing you to enact these scenarios in real life. They're fantasies, not wishes. For example, you might fantasize about things that you already know you don't want to do in real life—like sex with a stranger or your ex or a vampire. That's okay, and it's also sort of the point. Here is your chance to explore these sex acts without actually going through with them—unless you want to.

Romance and Erotica

The genre of erotic fiction has been around for centuries and is hotter than ever—double meaning intended. Reading something sexy can help us get in the mood to have sex, either with a partner or with ourselves. It can also get our fantasy thoughts spinning to enhance our solo session even more.

Audio Erotica

The world of erotic audio is exploding right now. This is a great option because it allows you to pop in your earbuds, lie back, and let all sorts of sexy content flow directly into your ears and mind. To many people, this feels more intimate and exciting than watching porn.

Ethical Porn

Most of the mainstream porn out there is made for penis owners by penis owners with little thought as to what vulva owners want or need—including the vulva owners that appear in the porn itself. Sometimes, the sex depicted in this type of porn can appear aggressive or violent. It certainly isn't meant to look realistic. Porn is entertainment, not documentary footage. It often shows the vulva owner having an orgasm after a few moments of penetrative sex, creating a completely unrealistic expectation, and it almost always ends with the penis owner (or owners) ejaculating. I've spoken to so many people who don't enjoy this type of porn and others who do enjoy it but still have mixed feelings because they know that it's exploitative and artificial.

Thankfully, there's a new trend in porn called ethical porn, which I'm really excited about. It shows inclusive, consensual, diverse, body-positive sex, and it's usually made by vulva owners using fair and safe production practices.

Lube

There is perhaps nothing that enhances pleasure more than lube. In fact, one of my dreams is a lube on every nightstand. Probably my most often repeated piece of advice is to add more lube! There are actually different types of lubes for different times. "Pre-lubes" have become more popular lately, especially those infused with CBD. These enhance blood flow and are meant to be applied ten to thirty minutes before climax. Water-based lubricants feel more natural and can be used with silicone or latex products. Plus, they don't stain and aren't sticky, but you may want to reapply during play. Silicone-based lubes are longer lasting, so they're best for marathon sessions or water play since they don't wash away. Oil-based lubes are great for erotic massages, but they aren't safe to use with condoms or sex toys made from rubber, PVC, or latex.

Sex Toys

Before we get into one of my favorite topics—sex toys—there are so many brands that I'm a huge fan of and many new pleasure products and accessories popping up all the time. Please check my website sexwithemily.com, or use the QR code in the back of the book for my top recommendations for every body part and occasion.

Sex toys have been marketed to vulvas for so long that many penis owners don't even realize that they can use them, too, but they are great aids to enhance everyone's pleasure.

If you're a penis owner who has difficulty getting or staying hard, you can use them to train your erections. Toys are excellent at promoting blood flow, which is exactly what the penis needs to maintain an erection. You can also use toys for the practice of building up a lot of sensation to your penis super quickly and then backing off right before you orgasm. This is called edging. Cycle through building up and then backing off for as long as you like. This can lead to a more intense orgasm. If you tend to orgasm before you'd like, toy stimulation is a great way to practice elongating your arousal.

Both vulva and penis owners have some nerve endings deep inside that are hard to reach with a hand (or even a penis during penetrative sex). So, toys are a fantastic way of leveling up your solo (or partnered) sessions. For an updated list of the brands I personally trust, check my website, sexwithemily.com.

First, let me bust a common misconception about vibrators. Some people are afraid that if they get used to using one, that they won't be able to have an orgasm with a partner. Our bodies do have muscle memories and remember how to orgasm if we always do it a certain way. If your routine never varies, then your muscle memory for other ways to climax could potentially stagnate. It's a good idea to stay in shape and work out your "muscles" so you can orgasm a few different ways.

Think of your solo sessions as cross-training. Mix it up. Use your hands sometimes and a vibrator during other times. It might take a bit longer to orgasm this way, but if you give yourself permission to spend ten or fifteen minutes exploring with plenty of lube and without any pressure to orgasm, you might discover new sensations and ways to orgasm that you've never experienced before.

There have been times when I felt I was relying too much on my go-to vibe because I used it in the same way on the same part of my body every time. So, I decided it was time to mix things up. This is when I learned to reconnect to my body without a toy, exploring different types of touch and arousal build. Then I added back in a different toy to mix up sensation.

Also, remember that different vibrators create different sensations. Explore with a variety of toys, and don't be afraid to throw in some for anal play, too, regardless of whether you have a vulva or a penis. There is a whole world of options out there to choose from for all body parts, at all price points, and with the ease of ordering online with delivery right to your door.

When choosing toys, avoid using toys made with rubber, vinyl, or PVC if you can, and opt instead for silicone, especially platinum cured, or materials that can be sterilized, like borosilicate glass or stainless steel.

Sex Toys

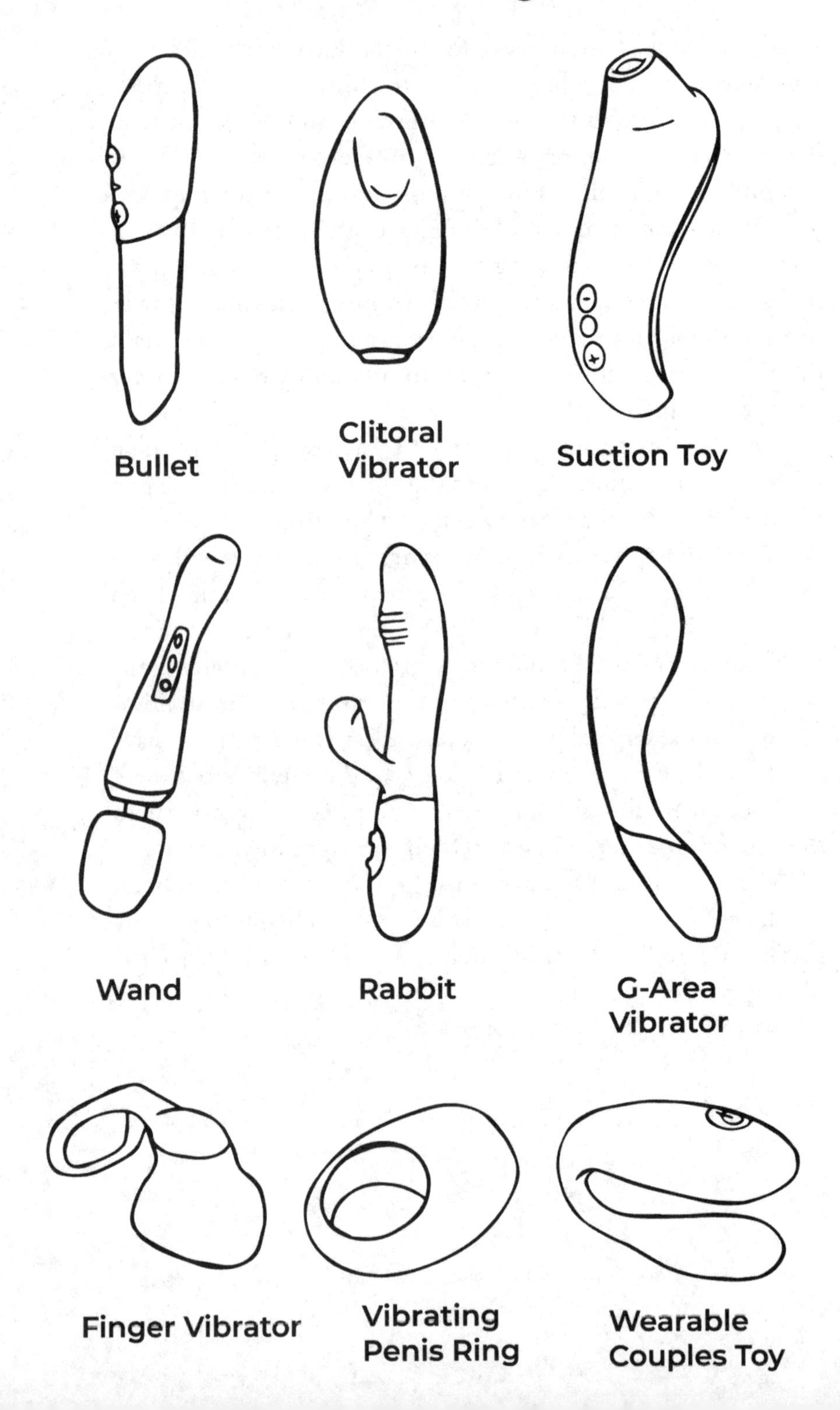
Bullet
Clitoral Vibrator
Suction Toy
Wand
Rabbit
G-Area Vibrator
Finger Vibrator
Vibrating Penis Ring
Wearable Couples Toy

Sex Toys

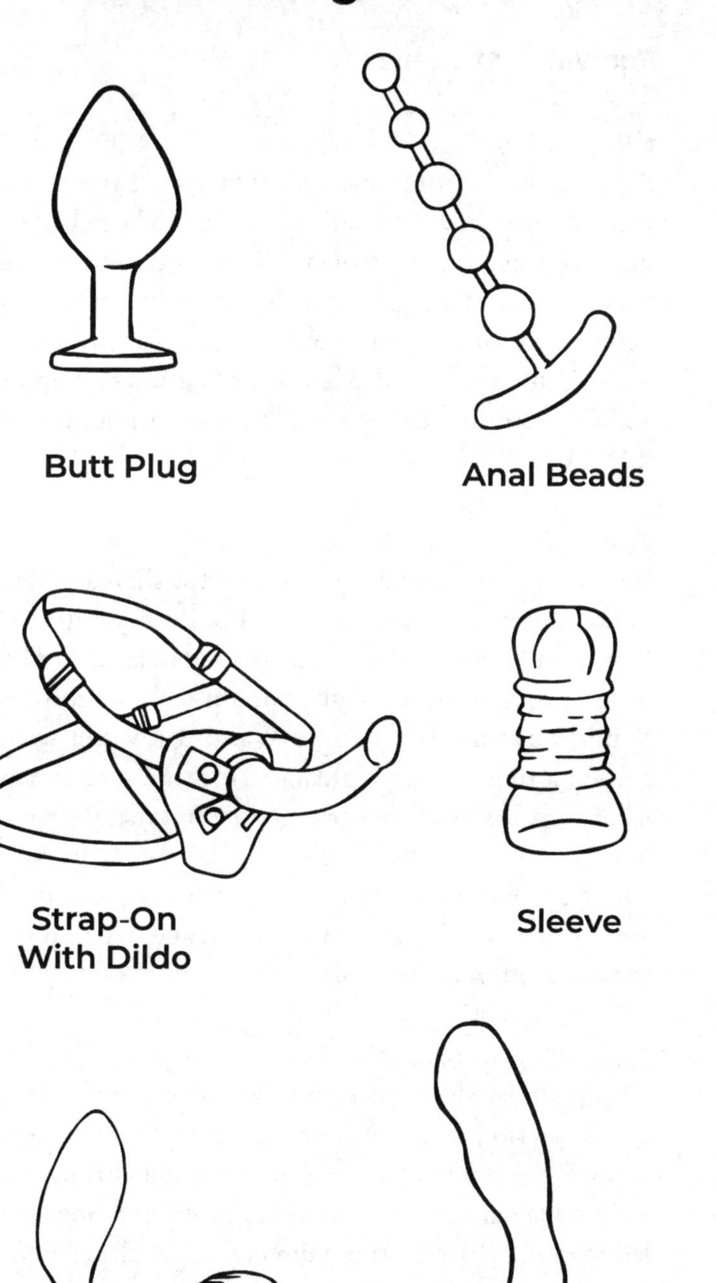
Butt Plug
Anal Beads
Strap-On
With Dildo
Sleeve
Prostate Vibrator
Prostate Stimulator

For Vulva Owners:

Clitoral Vibes

If you're just starting out with vibrators, I recommend a bullet vibe because they are small, powerful, and can be less intimidating than some other products. They tend to have pointed tips to make them easier to target different body parts. Bullet vibes are best for external use on the clitoris, vulva, and nipples. Finger-mount vibrators are also great for beginners. Slip one right on and they promise to get the job done without being so powerful that they'll knock you off the bed.

Power Vibes

Wands are larger and more powerful than smaller, handheld vibes and can be used as overall body massagers. The Magic Wand is all-powerful, so if you're used to a small vibrator, you're in for a real thrill. Though it might feel like too much at first! When I got my first Magic Wand, I loved it so much that I drilled a hole in my nightstand for the wire to run through. That way, it was always plugged in and ready to go. They now have a cordless rechargeable model, so your nightstand is safe. There are also dual stimulation power vibes like the Rabbit that are designed to provide both internal and external stimulation—these are often called "rabbits."

Suction Toys and Air Pulsation

This is a relatively new class of sex toys that are designed to use gentle suction or air, mimicking the best oral sex of your life. They focus solely on stimulating the clit through air-powered technology and pulsation and they provide indirect clitoral stimulation rather than the more direct contact placed with other toys.

Anal Toys

To experiment with anal stimulation as you masturbate I recommend starting with a butt plug. Start with a smaller size first and make sure it has a flared base that is wider than the part that goes inside you so it doesn't slip down into your anal cavity. That's an emergency room visit that no one wants to make. As your muscles adjust, you can try larger plugs to create deeper, more intense sensations. These come with vibrating and non-vibrating options.

For Penis Owners:

Sleeves/Strokers

Slip one on, add lube, and you'll find a new twist on a familiar experience. Most are made of elastomer sleeves with internal nubs and grooves that simulate penetrative or oral sex. Some of the sleeves are intended for single use, and some can be washed out and reused. In recent years, this product category has grown to include vibrations and suction to stimulate the frenulum and the entire shaft.

Vibrating Rings (aka Cock Rings)

Worn around the penis—or sometimes dildos! These rings can have built-in vibrators or leave space for a bullet vibe. This is fun for partner play, too. A penis ring stimulates the perineum, the sensitive area between the balls and the anus that indirectly stimulates the prostate. And positioned accordingly, the vibrating motor can come in contact with the clitoris during penetrative sex, which can enhance pleasure for everyone!

Prostate Stimulators

While butt plugs are fun for vulva or penis owners, these toys are specifically designed to stimulate the sensitive prostate. They often have a curve that makes it easier to contact the prostate. Remember that they need to have a wide flared base to keep them from slipping into the rectum.

Mutual Masturbation

Masturbation is giving yourself pleasure alone. Partner sex is sharing pleasure together. Mutual masturbation is the best of both worlds.

Practically speaking, mutual masturbation means that you and your partner are together while you touch yourself and they touch themselves. This is also a fantastic option for anyone who's in a long-distance relationship or who travels frequently, or if you're healing from an infection and want to keep your body and fluids to yourself. You can engage in mutual masturbation over the phone or Zoom or even in the same room!

Mutual masturbation is one of my favorite activities for a few reasons. First of all, watching my partner turn themselves on is incredibly arousing. I'm guaranteed to have an orgasm because I know what it takes for me to experience one. And best of all, it's educational.

As you watch your partner please themselves, you will learn so much about how they like to be touched. No one is a bigger expert in your pleasure than you—and the same thing goes for your partner. Why not learn from the best?

Sometimes, I like to narrate so that my partners understand why I'm touching myself a certain way. "Look at how my clitoris responds when I do this," I tell them. "Isn't that cool how it gets bigger?" More often than not, they are super turned on and into it. I swear they are tempted to grab a notepad and write it all down.

If you feel nervous about this idea, I promise that when your partner sees you touch yourself with confidence, they will be entranced by it. Hypnotized, even. Whether it's watching a partner excel on the field, stage, boardroom, or bedroom, it's a turn-on to see them shine. Mutual masturbation is an opportunity to show your partner your sexual confidence and mastery and to behold theirs.

If you're not sure how to bring this up with your partner, try saying, "I'd love to see how you touch yourself...and for you to watch me, too." Or try turning your pleasure into a game. Make it fun! Say to your partner, "Let's see how turned on we can make ourselves without touching each other for ten minutes." Set a timer, and then see how it feels to build sexual tension without being able to touch each other.

Mutual masturbation can include toys or no toys, touching each other and yourselves, or strictly just touching yourselves, and so many other fun enhancements that you can choose. The most basic and popular position is for you and your partner to lie on the bed next to each other (or sit up) as you individually touch yourselves with your fingers or a favorite toy. As you each get stimulated, try moving to face each other and add some intimate eye contact.

If you want more of a physical connection, try getting on top of your partner while touching yourself. They can also touch themselves while you straddle them. A nice variation here is to turn around and lean back against your partner. Feel the weight of your bodies touching one another as you touch yourself.

To take it even further, eliminate the rule of not touching each other, and take turns physically stimulating each other while you masturbate. If your partner has a penis, try licking their balls while they masturbate, or see how they respond to a little anal play (with permission first). If your partner has a vulva, how do they react when you squeeze their nipples? Or find out how they feel about you inserting a butt plug while they use a vibrator against their clitoris.

We have so many places to explore and experience pleasure, the sky is truly the limit here! And if you both want to finish your session with penetrative or another form of sex, go for it. Think of mutual masturbation as one more tool in your arsenal of all-around pleasure enhancers.

Meditate. Masturbate. Manifest.

Speaking of tools in your personal pleasure arsenal, this is another one of my favorites. It's a powerful practice that has the potential to not only give you more pleasure, but also to radically change your life. This is exactly what it has done for me.

Many people who believe in alchemy, or a magical process of transformation, also believe that orgasms are a powerful tool to help you create your desires. This has led to a "sex magic" movement of people who use their orgasms to help them manifest their dream lives.

"Meditate. Masturbate. Manifest." is my version of this movement. I use this as a morning ritual to start my day on the right note while being intentional about my goals. I start with a meditation to clear my thoughts, focus on my breath, and set my intention. This is a book about sex, not meditation, but if you don't already have a meditation practice, I highly encourage you to start one. In addition to all sorts of other benefits, it's a great tool to help you become more mindful and to shift into a more sensual state of mind.

Next, I indulge in some mindful masturbation while focusing on my pleasure, all of the sensations that I'm feeling, and my breath. When done right, mindful masturbation is a meditation in practice. After I have an orgasm, I take a moment to be present in the afterglow and imagine sending powerful energy toward my goals. Sometimes, I spend a few minutes visualizing or journaling about them coming true and imagining how it would feel. The number one rule of manifestation is that if you can imagine and feel something happening, it is already done.

This practice is a beautiful way of expanding your high-vibrating, blissful, post-orgasm moment of self-love and self-care into all areas of your life. Try incorporating the "Meditate. Masturbate. Manifest." practice into your days, and soon you will be creating a more pleasurable life for yourself while discovering your vast and unlimited potential.

Whether you're partnered or single, the most important sexual relationship that you will ever have is your sexual relationship with yourself. By exploring your sexuality on your own, you will grow in all of the Sex IQ pillars and make any partnered sex that you choose to have far more pleasurable. It's incredibly empowering to know what you want in bed and to be able to give this information to a partner. Which brings me to our next chapter...

4

Communication Is Lubrication:

How to Talk to Your Partner(s) About Your Sexual Needs

I've always thought of myself as a good communicator. Ever since I was young, I've loved talking to people and learning all about them, and long before I started *Sex with Emily*, I noticed that people had a tendency to open up and confide in me. It didn't matter where I was—at an event, a coffee shop, or in line at the grocery store—I could talk to anyone who crossed my path and really connect with them.

It was the same way with my sexual partners. Whenever I was dating someone, I felt super connected to them. We talked all the time about our days, our jobs, and our greatest hopes and dreams.

Then, as the relationship progressed, conflicts and issues inevitably popped up—some that were related to sex and others that had nothing to do with sex at all. And while I was great at chatting it up when things were going well, I had no idea how to communicate through conflict. When I felt smothered, I didn't know how to tell my partner that I needed more space. When I felt sexually unsatisfied and needed more of something that I wasn't getting, I didn't know how to request it.

It turned out that all of that talk, talk, talking had done nothing for my ability to really communicate. And my relationships could not survive without the communication skills that I'm going to teach you in this chapter. When unspoken conflict led to blame and resentment and a lack of collaboration, the relationship was eventually doomed.

I now know that, like so many of my past sex and relationship issues, this was mainly a cultural problem and not an Emily problem. We're not exactly taught how to communicate with our partners about sex. And nobody tells us that most of the sexual problems in our relationships have nothing to do with sex and everything to do with communication.

Let me say that again one more time—most of the sexual problems in our relationships have nothing to do with sex and everything to do with communication.

The silence and shame around sex keeps it shrouded in mystery, so it seems simpler, less messy, and less fraught to just avoid the subject completely. We try to convince ourselves that maybe the sex will magically get better or that maybe sex isn't that important after all. I remember a friend once telling me that she'd had enough sex with her husband of fifteen years, so why did she have to work on it?

Most of us feel uncomfortable talking about sex because we have no idea that it's a normal thing to talk about. We don't see many healthy models of people talking about sex in our culture, so we assume that it's unnecessary. We think that great sex should just happen. Our partners should intuitively know how to satisfy us. If it's not happening, we believe the "spark" just isn't there and that it's unfixable.

If you learn one thing from this book, I hope it's this: it's a complete and total myth that great sex should just happen automatically and that talking about it will rob it of its magic. The truth is that *communication is the magic.*

True intimacy requires vulnerability. And good sex—I'm talking about really good sex—requires intimacy. When we hold ourselves back from telling our partners what we want and need to feel maximum pleasure, we are shortchanging ourselves of that pleasure itself, and we're keeping ourselves and our partners from experiencing the full depths of our connection.

I always say that communication is lubrication because next to actual lube, it's the number one thing that is going to improve your sex life. Seriously. The more you talk about sex with your partners, the more comfortable you are going to be talking about sex with your partners. And the more comfortable you are talking about sex with your partners, the better your sex is going to be. On and on in a virtuous cycle of healthy communication and great sex.

Notice that I said "healthy communication." Like anything in relationships, there is a way of talking about sex that increases intimacy and collaboration between you and your partner and a way of talking about sex that does more harm than good. A lot of people think that communicating with their partners about sex means shouting, "Do this! Not like that!" Worse yet, we assume that if our partner has to give us any feedback at all it must mean that we're terrible in bed. That's not the kind of communication that I'm talking about.

Instead, I want you to have ongoing open, judgment-free conversations about sex from a place of love and mutual respect. Ideally, you should start having these conversations early in your relationships, even before you get naked with your partner with the shared goal of connection and pleasure. This is the only way to know whether or not you're dating someone who has a growth mindset about sex, meaning that it's something they're willing to learn more about and explore together in collaboration.

Most of the time, people want to be good lovers, but they don't know how to challenge their limiting beliefs around sex or even realize that these beliefs exist or aren't facts. I can't stress how important it is to know whether or not your partner is willing to challenge these assumptions before you get serious, especially if you're considering walking down the aisle and promising to stay together for life.

I remember speaking to a gentleman who told me that his wife of thirty years never once gave him a blow job, leaving him dissatisfied. Her mom had told her when she was young that good girls don't give blow jobs, and the conversation was closed before it ever opened. Had she been willing to look at her sexual history and challenge this messaging, they could have turned their sex life around, but with a closed mindset, the conversation was off-limits, and blow jobs were off the table. This man loved his wife, but he never had the sex life that he wanted and probably could have had.

It's just as important to continue the conversation around sex throughout your relationship as it is to start early. This is not something that you should talk about once or when there's a major problem or you have a big request. Talking about sex should become a normal, frequent part of your life. By talking about it regularly, you'll create a culture of healthy sex communication within your partnership. This will help you intentionally create the sex life you want and make it so much easier to bring up issues when they inevitably come up.

Start by surrounding yourselves with sex-positive and sex-curious voices. Clear out and replace that old sex messaging that was negative, fear based, and steeped in shame. Choose at least three sex-positive voices to bring into your life. They can be movies or TV shows that depict sex in a healthy or educational light, or social media accounts, books, or podcasts from trusted sex educators. (Check out the reference section in the back of the book for some great ideas.) These resources will give you a new vocabulary for your sex life.

Commit to engaging with at least one of these voices each week, and then share what you've learned with your partner. Even better, watch the shows and listen to the podcasts together, share the social media posts, or read aloud from the books. I love it when people tell me that they played my podcast in the car with their partner and it turned their sex life around.

Adding any of these voices to the world of your relationship will help liberate your own conversations around sex. Simply getting used to listening to other people talk about sex will normalize sex communication. This will help you feel more comfortable with the idea of talking about it yourself. You are literally learning a new language here, so the more you hear it and use it in action, the more skillful you will become.

This is important because when the topic of sex comes up, many of us immediately shift into a sympathetic or stressed state. We feel threatened. Either we're afraid of how our partner is going to react to what we have to say, or we're scared of what our partner might say to us. I compare this to someone telling you "We need to talk." Of course, we immediately shift into a stressed state just upon hearing those words.

To make it less stressful, ease your way into talking about sex. A conversation about sex—and sex itself—is always better when it starts off slowly. Try testing the waters with a preliminary conversation about having a conversation about sex. Keep this preliminary conversation lighthearted and positive, and make sure to put your partner at ease by making it clear that this isn't going to be some big confrontation. Let them know that you want to continue to explore and grow together because you feel so connected to them.

Or you can always blame me. Tell your partner, "Dr. Emily suggests that all couples talk about their sex lives. What do you say? Want to give it a try?" Make it fun and flirty so it doesn't feel like yet another chore or obligation. If your partner seems uncomfortable, agree to table it and try bringing it up again another time. Be patient and understanding. This is about their own comfort, not about you.

If your partner is receptive to the idea of talking about your sex life, you can continue on to the real conversation right then and there or agree to bring it up at a better time. So, when is the best time?

The Three *T*s

When the time comes for the actual conversation, give yourself the best possible chance of having a healthy and productive (and maybe even fun) dialogue by following my Three *T*s for successful sexual communication: Timing, Tone, and Turf.

Timing

Often, *when* you talk about something important is just as important—or even more so—than your actual words. It's best to have this conversation when you're both in a parasympathetic state—relaxed, energized, and at ease. The conversation will go nowhere fast if either of you is in a sympathetic state of stress. In this state, you'll be so much more likely to be reactive and defensive instead of able to listen and respond calmly and with an open mind.

To work with your nervous system to time this conversation perfectly, remember this easy acronym: HALT. If either of you is hungry, angry, lonely, or tired, you're much more likely to react poorly to the conversation. If either of you is in HALT mode, save the talk for another time. It's not worth pushing forward with a planned conversation if the timing is off.

Tone

In any conversation, but especially one about sex, make sure to lead with curiosity and compassion rather than blame or criticism, which are both conversation stoppers. It's important here to get curious. Ask questions, and if your partner says "I don't know" in response, that's okay. It probably means that they actually don't know and aren't intentionally withholding information. Remember, you are exploring together, not badgering the witness.

In addition to asking questions, use lots of "I feel" statements and the words "we" and "us" so that it's clear to your partner that you're in this together. Try to avoid words like "never" and "always." Saying things like "You never go down on me," or "You always expect me to initiate" sound more like accusations than conversation starters. Better options would be "I get so turned on when you go down on me," or "I think it would be so hot if you initiated sex."

It's also essential that you listen just as much as you talk! Practice active listening, which involves responding in an intentional way that shows the other person they've been heard. One communication style that I especially like is called Imago Relationship Therapy, or IRT, which was developed by Harville Hendrix and Helen LaKelly Hunt. IRT uses mirroring, validation, and empathy to turn conflict into compassion. Each partner takes a turn making a statement, and then the other partner repeats it back to confirm that they heard what was said. Then they switch roles.

Let's say that one partner says they want to receive more oral. Instead of responding defensively—"How dare you accuse me of not giving you enough oral?"—the Imago response would be "What I hear you saying is that you desire more oral. Is that right?" The first partner might confirm that is what they said. Then the other partner might get upset and say, "That's so unfair! It feels like you always accuse me of doing things wrong!

Nothing I do is ever good enough." The other partner would say, "I hear you saying that you feel I accuse you of many things and that this feels unfair." And so on.

This can feel awkward and tedious at first, but there is a good reason behind this method. When we really slow down and listen to what our partner is saying and repeat it back, they feel truly heard. Plus, they have an opportunity to correct us if we misinterpret something they've said. This forces us to hear exactly what they are saying instead of coloring their statements with our own interpretations.

Finally, this method doesn't allow us to argue with our partner's feelings, which is a losing battle. It's not helpful to tell your partner that you disagree with their interpretation of what happened and how it impacted their feelings. Whether we agree with it or not, we come to understand our partner's unique reality.

No matter what method you use, the less reactive and the more mindful you can be during this conversation, the more likely you will be to create win-win situations by arriving at a mutual understanding.

When Conversations Turn Ugly

In some relationships, there is a lot of water under the bridge that makes it difficult to have an open and honest conversation about sex or any aspect of the relationship. If you or your partner has a lot of resentment built up and the two of you can't have this conversation without blaming or criticizing or becoming reactive or defensive, consider working with a therapist to work through some of those issues. With help, you will be able to start communicating about sex and other relationship issues in healthier ways.

It's very common for one partner to refuse to talk about sex and be unwilling to go to therapy. Unfortunately, many people don't discover that their partner is so resistant to these things until there's a crisis in the relationship. This is exactly why I encourage you to start talking about sex in the beginning.

If you find yourself in this position, follow the Three *T*s steps to ask your partner why they don't want to go to therapy. They may have had a bad experience in the past, feel uncomfortable sharing such personal details with a stranger, or worry that the therapist will "take sides." If they absolutely refuse, it's important for you to go to therapy on your own and start to do your own work. This will help you develop the strength and self-knowledge that you'll need to take the next step, whatever that may be. Perhaps your partner will see your growth and want to join you, or they might stay stuck. Either way, you can only control yourself and do what you need to do to keep growing and evolving.

Turf

I cannot stress this enough—do not have this conversation in the bedroom. You might assume that the bedroom is the perfect place to talk about sex, but do yourself a favor and save the bedroom as a sacred space for sleeping and sex itself. This will help you get more of both!

Instead, talk about sex somewhere neutral that isn't charged with sexual expectation. It should be somewhere that is relaxing for you and your partner: on the living room couch, outside on the patio or while taking a walk, at the kitchen table over your weekend coffee, or in the car during a road trip. Cars and walks work well for many people because you're not forced to make eye contact while you talk. This makes it easier for some people to engage in a vulnerable conversation.

Types of Sex Talks

Maybe you already know exactly what you want to say to your partner about sex, or maybe you just want to open up this conversation and see where it goes. Either way, take a moment to think about your goals for the conversation. Are there specific requests that you want to make or topics that you want to bring up? Are you curious about your partner's thoughts and feelings about sex? Do you want to know whether or not they are satisfied and if there's anything new or different that they want to try?

Depending on exactly what you want to get out of the conversation, I have specific tools to help. Here are a few different types of sex talks based on what you want to communicate, along with my best practices:

Giving Feedback

It can be very difficult to give your partner delicate feedback about their performance in bed. But this is often necessary for the sake of your long-term mutual pleasure. Once you start communicating honestly about sex, there are likely going to be times when you have to tell your partner that something they are doing or not doing—or even something about them—is turning you off. Yikes.

My go-to solution for giving delicate feedback is the **Compliment Sandwich**. This is a disarming way of sharing constructive feedback by nestling it delicately in between compliments, which of course we all love to receive. The Compliment Sandwich starts with an affirmation, moves to feedback, and then ends with more affirmation. Simple and effective.

Maybe you have a partner who sweats a lot. By the end of the day they have distracting body odor, and you want them to shower before sex. You could say, "I really love your body. It's so sexy. I know we just want to rip each other's clothes off the minute we get home, but it'd be even sexier if we took a shower together before we get down to business. I want us to feel clean before we get dirty."

Many people, especially vulva owners, want their partners to slow down. You could say, "I love how much you desire me, and that you just want to ravage me. It's so hot. I'd love it if you teased me a bit more and we took our time so I get nice and wet. It'll make things even hotter and feel so much better for both of us, if that's possible."

Or if you want to get more adventurous, you could say, "I've never felt so connected to a partner in my life. We're so in sync, and I feel so safe with you. What would you think about experimenting with some new toys or positions? With our connection being what it is, I can only imagine what would happen if we mixed it up."

As you can see, the Compliment Sandwich is gold for sensitive feedback, especially when paired with the three *T*s. Of course, you can customize your sandwich. This is not a one-size-fits-all situation! Just make sure that the compliments you give your partner are just as sincere as your requests. When you express your desires in loving and thoughtful ways, your partner is way more likely to hear you and be responsive to what you're saying.

Another tactic that I like to use for giving feedback is what I call **Show and Tell**. Unlike other sex talks, this one does happen in the bedroom in real time, turning a less than ideal situation into a teachable moment.

Let's say that you're feeling frustrated because your partner jumps right into penetrative sex as soon as you start kissing, with little to no foreplay. You're not even fully aroused before your partner is pounding away. As I said above, this is a common complaint among vulva owners. So, why not use a hands-on approach?

The next time you're kissing, use it as an opportunity to show your partner exactly what you want. Give your partner some slow, sensual kisses on the neck. Then tease them over their pants or give them oral nice and slow with lots of eye contact. Then tell your partner, "If you explored me like this before we have sex, it would really turn me on."

With Show and Tell, feedback becomes experiential. You

allow your partner to feel and experience the kind of sex you want. Hopefully, they'll take their turn and you'll discover the kind of sex they want, and find that there's plenty of overlap.

Your Greatest Hits

This type of sex talk helps you improve your future sex life by pinpointing what's worked for you as a couple in the past. To have this talk, simply start reminiscing about some of the most memorable sex you've had together. "Remember that one time...?"

Explain exactly what made it so hot for you. What state of mind were you in when it happened? Were you in a different location or position, or was there something else that made you feel extra connected and turned on?

Maybe your most memorable times together were early in the relationship when things were new. This is very common. It's called the honeymoon phase for a reason! During this time, everything is novel. You've never kissed this person before or seen them naked or had sex with them in this position, and it's all so exciting.

After a while, things naturally shift into a more familiar stage. This is often comforting and safe, but is in direct opposition to being hot and new. It makes sense for you to crave the type of sex you had in those early days. So, how can you bring some novelty back into the bedroom? Try something you've never done before, have sex in a new location, or indulge in some sexy role-play. The idea is to leverage what you've learned about your desire from pinpointing your greatest hits.

Another popular greatest hit is vacation sex. On vacation, you're apart from the stresses of everyday life, and you feel free and relaxed. Plus, you're probably more well rested and have more time to explore in bed. This is the perfect recipe for hot sex.

If this is you, think about how can you replicate this vacation vibe when you're at home. Maybe send the kids away for the weekend, or keep your date night super chill and relaxing, or even shake things up by going to a local hotel just for the night. These small things can make a big difference.

To have this conversation, you can either bring up one of your favorite sexual memories and let it flow naturally from there, or make it more of a game. Each of you can write down your top three sexual experiences together and then compare lists. Then see how you can leverage the information that you glean from your lists to keep making your sex life better.

The Sexual Bucket List

Most of us have a few sexual activities that we'd like to try one day, but we haven't gotten around to or we haven't felt comfortable bringing up to a partner. Yet. Talking about your Sexual Bucket List is a great way to get imaginative about your sex life and become co-conspirators with your partner.

Again, you can start a conversation—"Is there anything that you've always wanted to try in the bedroom?" or "Do you know what I've always fantasized about doing, just once..." Or make it a game. Have each of you write down your top three "bucket list" items and then trade lists.

Maybe you'll discover that you've both always been curious about threesomes or that your partner is more open to a little bondage than you ever would have thought. Even if there's not much overlap between your lists, taking the time to learn about your partner's desires and your own is one of the most important things that you can do to move the needle on your mutual pleasure.

Remember to be patient and consistent with these conversations. They will get easier over time, and eventually you won't have to remember to have these talks because they'll be built into the framework of your relationship. Along the way, you'll see your sex life turn from a problem you need to fix to an area that you can keep evolving and growing together.

Yes! No! Maybe?

When we go to a restaurant, we're handed a menu. We know what the options are. But we're never handed a menu for sex. As a result, most of us have no idea about all of the many exciting options that are available to us in the bedroom.

You can think of this game as your menu of sexual options. Label each one with a "yes," "no," or "maybe." Simply doing this will help you learn so much about yourself. Even better, sharing your list with your partner and taking a look at theirs is a great way of expressing your needs, boundaries, curiosities, and desires in a fun, nonjudgmental, and nonshaming way. Just as important, this is a fun way of learning more about your partner. How wonderful to discover that you've both been craving bathing together or a little light bondage!

There is also a lot of magic in the "maybes." Often, a Pleasure Thief like shame is the one thing keeping a "maybe" from becoming a "yes." Once you clear that shame away, you'll have more "yesses" on your list and more opportunities to scream, "YES!"

This list is just a jumping-off point, and you can either use it as its own conversation starter or to inform your Sexual Bucket List. You can also download this list on my website sexwithemily.com and print it out so you can take notes.

Anal sex
Anal rimming (giving/receiving)
Anal toys (giving/receiving)

Biting (giving/receiving)
Blindfolds (on you or on your partner)
Bathing together
Bondage (giving/receiving)
Caressing (giving/receiving)
Choking (giving/receiving)
Compliments (giving/receiving)
Cuckolding (see page 262 for more on this)
Cuddling
Climaxing together
Deep throating (giving/receiving)
Deep breathing together
Dirty talk (giving/receiving)
Dressing up in costume
Edging (you or your partner)
Eye contact
Face Sitting (giving/receiving)
Fingering (giving/receiving)
Fisting (giving/receiving)
Flirting (giving/receiving)
Food play
Foot massage (giving/receiving)
G-area stimulation (giving/receiving)
Gags (on you or your partner)
Genital massage (giving/receiving)
Group sex
Hair pulling (giving/receiving)
Hand jobs (giving/receiving)
Handcuffs (on you or your partner)
Homemade porn
Humiliation (giving/receiving)
Hot wax massage candle (giving/receiving)
Lap dance (giving/receiving)
Licking (giving/receiving)

Making out
Mutual masturbation
Massaging inner thighs (giving/receiving)
Neck kissing (giving/receiving)
Nipple play (giving/receiving)
Oral sex (giving/receiving)
Orgasm denial (you or your partner)
Phone sex
Period sex
Penis rings
Penis worship (giving/receiving)
Post-sex shower together
Prostate stimulation (giving/receiving)
Role-play
Sexting
Sex games
Sex parties
Sex outside
Sex toy play (giving/receiving)
Sex toy shopping
Slow sex
Spanking (giving/receiving)
Squirting
Strap-on play (giving/receiving)
Striptease (giving/receiving)
Swapping
Swinging
Tantric sex
Threesomes
Temperature play (giving/receiving)
Watching porn together
Wearing lingerie
Vulva worship (giving/receiving)

The Sexual State of the Union

My goal is for sex to become something that you talk about in your relationships with the same level of comfort, normalcy, and intention as planning a vacation or where to go on a fun night out. With open communication and the right mindset you can create the sex life of your dreams. To get there, it's important to have a clear understanding of what's currently working in your sex life for both you and your partner and what isn't. The Sexual State of the Union is a great way to get this conversation started.

This can be a fun conversation to have on a date night and it can even serve as a form of conversational foreplay. I suggest aiming to have a Sexual State of the Union once a month. Remember that if your partner says "I don't know" to a lot of these questions, they probably just haven't yet identified their turn-ons. Rather than going in expecting your partner to know every one of their kinks, fantasies, fetishes, and desires, start with your own vulnerability, stay curious, and keep the conversation light and flirty. Remember, this should be fun, not stressful!

These questions will get you going, but as time goes on and you have more of these conversations, feel free to tailor the questions to your relationship.

- What are you enjoying about our sex life right now?
- What would you like to see more of in our sex life?
- What's something new you'd like to try?
- When you think about the hottest sex we could ever have, what does it look like?
- Where are we when that fantasy happens?
- What can I do more of to make sex satisfying for you?
- What's your favorite memory of sex we've had as a couple?

- What was a moment recently when you felt super turned on?
- May I share something I'd like more of during sex?
- When we're having sex, what's your favorite part about it?

The Sexual Fantasy Elevator Pitch

An elevator pitch is used when you want to sell someone on an idea. It's a short, punchy statement that summarizes what you're selling, and it's called an elevator pitch because you can complete it in the time between the elevator doors closing and then reopening when you reach your floor. It's all about keeping your pitch short and sweet.

In this case, you're pitching a sexual fantasy. The trick here is to quickly communicate what you want and why, all while letting your partner know how it can be hot for them, too. Once you make your pitch, don't say anything else. It can be tempting to keep blabbering as a means of explaining, but hold back and give them a beat to process while they formulate their response.

Here are some examples of Sexual Fantasy Elevator Pitches:

"I love how sensual we are in bed. I've been thinking about how hot it would be for you to blindfold me. If you take away my sight, I'll be able to feel your touch on my body even more strongly. Do you want to try it?" Notice how this explains how doing what you want will improve the sex for both of you. It invites your partner to explore with you in collaboration.

"You're such a sexy lover. It almost makes me want to watch you with someone else. Have you ever fantasized about having a threesome? I'd only be down if you are, but if the idea turns you on, I'd love to explore it together." Notice how this one frames the fantasy in the context of your partner's pleasure. It's not just about what you want, but what you both want.

"I so appreciate the fact that we keep our sex life adventurous. I know we haven't done it before, but I'd love to experiment with anal sex. Do you want to try and see if it feels good? With the right prep, I think we both might love it." Notice how this makes the fantasy about a journey the two of you are taking together. Remember, it's a collaboration!

Once you get used to making your pitches directly and succinctly, you can take this a step further by actually making your pitch in an elevator. Turn it into a sexy game. Create a rule that anytime the two of you find yourselves alone in an elevator, one of you has to make a Sexual Fantasy Elevator Pitch. Then on the next elevator ride, it's your partner's turn. I promise you will never be bored in an elevator again!

Get Your Flirt On

Flirting is a great way to build sexual tension through communication. So, it only makes sense to add a bit of flirtation to all of our conversations about sex. When we flirt, we're using curiosity, humor, empathy, and a sense of playfulness, all in service of the other person. It's a way of putting the spotlight on them. No wonder we all find flirting to be so irresistibly hot.

Flirting is not about getting what we want right now in the moment. Rather, it's a sexy sort of restraint, where your behavior is suggestive (not explicit), and your vibe is patient (not desperate). When we are flirting, we are present and focused on our partners, but we are intentionally putting off our pleasure and allowing desire to build as we stoke those flames. The best flirts know how to invite others into their playful space, where there's a bit of a push and pull between the two of you.

Ask yourself how you can flirt with your partner more. This is one thing that so often goes out the window over time in our relationships. Adding flirtation back into the mix can bring back sexual tension, enhance our sex lives in general, and make all of our conversations about sex that much more fun.

One great way to flirt is over text—or sext. Many people get sexting all wrong and suddenly start sending explicit messages or even nude pics to their partners. But a great sext builds anticipation, instead. It's all about creating sexual tension via your phone.

Before you start sexting, it's important to make sure you have consent. It's also a good idea to agree to keep your sexting private, so those messages or pics don't end up anywhere you don't want them to. Try something along the lines of, "If it's okay with you, I'd love to take this party to WhatsApp," (if you prefer a secure messaging option), or, "I can't wait to do this, but first, can we agree to delete afterward?"

Another quick pregame tip: make sure your phone settings are conducive to this endeavor. Say you get a nude, you save it, and it automatically uploads to your kid's iPad? Please don't let that happen. While you're at it, go ahead and double-check that you've cued up "Dan" and not "Dad." Let's not accidentally sext our parents.

Okay, you've gotten consent, laid down the ground rules, your phone is good, and now it's time for action. Yes! For your opening sext, I recommend something playful and open-ended. The classic "What are you wearing right now?" is always a popular option, next to "Can I tell you a secret?" What you're doing here is building up the sexual tension and energy by flirting. Keep things a little cheeky at first before you get to the fireworks.

Keep warming things up by describing a fantasy that involves the other person. This can be the "secret" you wanted to tell them. Something like "I can't stop thinking about putting my hand in your pants and feeling you get hard." Or "Remember when you pinned me to the wall? That really turned me on. I can't wait for you to do that again."

While I'm all for being present, this is a good time to draw inspiration from sex you've had with this person in the past and/or sex you imagine having with them in the future. "I can't stop thinking about how hot it was to look down at you as you climaxed," or "I can't wait to see you on top of me while I grab your hips and make you moan."

Remember, this is all about building anticipation. One of the best parts of sexting is watching the other person type while wondering what they're going to say next. So, draw it out! Let's deconstruct my example above: "I can't stop thinking about putting my hand in your pants and feeling you get hard."

Broken down into bite-sized, sexy bits, you can write it like this:

"I can't stop thinking about..."

"...putting my hand in your pants..."

"...and feeling you get hard."

Cute, right? Try this easy technique when you want to draw things out a little more, making the other person wait in the most painful, erotic way possible.

When you're ready to move on, it's always hot to tell your partner that you went shopping—for sex stuff, not groceries. Toys, lingerie, condoms, you name it. Try, "I just got some flavored lube...any ideas about who I should lick it off of?" (Hint: send a little pic of said item, for extra excitement. I dare them not to heart it.)

You may or may not be ready to send a nude pic. It's fine if you don't want to, but if you do, let's stick with our striptease analogy and increase the heat little by little. Before sending a full frontal, try something more suggestive at first, like a pic with your underwear on or your hand covering yourself strategically... If you don't ever feel comfortable sending a full-blown nude, that's okay, too.

If the other person is up for it, maybe they'll return the favor. The most important thing is that you're both having fun! Nothing about this should feel forced. And don't forget to tell them the effect they're having on you. Sexting, like all types of flirting, is part performance, part conversation. And we all enjoy positive reinforcement. So, let your partner know how turned on you're getting from all of the sexy things they're saying. A simple, "You're killing me," or even, "You're really good at this," can go a long way.

All of these sexting tips can translate just as easily to in-person flirting. Never stop seducing your partner, no matter how long you've been together. Above all else, this shows your partner that you still want them, which is a huge turn-on in and of itself. Even the most difficult and awkward of conversations can be made sexier and more fun with the help of a little flirting.

Consent and Boundaries

When I was younger, I spent years thinking that it was rude or even mean to stop sex once it got started. I believed that penis owners could suffer from "blue balls" and that it was a real, debilitating condition. (Heads-up—it's not.) I felt that I owed it to them to finish what we'd started, so I did. There were countless times when I wasn't saying no wholeheartedly, but I wasn't saying yes with gusto, either.

The advice that I wish I could give to my younger self and to anyone in any sexual situation would be to listen to your body. Things become very clear when you take a moment and ask yourself, "Is this a full-bodied YES or a full-bodied NO?" There is very little wiggle room between "Meh, my body is lukewarm on this idea at best," and "HELL, YES, I AM FEELING IT!"

Part of being embodied is tuning in to these signals to make sexual decisions. This is a practice that you can fine-tune over time, and when you do, it will be so much easier to tap into your true wants and desires. This is a powerful way of building self-knowledge.

Now I know that if my body isn't saying "Hell, yes" then it's a "Hell, no." Unless the sex is fully your choice and it's something that you're doing for the pleasure of it, then you absolutely do not need to consent to it. End of story!

Of course, it can be hard to say no in the moment. Besides

blue balls, when I was younger, I worried that saying no would hurt the other person's feelings or make them stop liking me. Ever the people pleaser! As I became more embodied, I found it easier to listen to my body, and you will likely experience the same thing and find it easier to start saying yes to what you want and no to what you don't want.

Sometimes things escalate really fast, and we just need a beat to check in with ourselves and make sure this is something we want. I find that the easiest way to do this is to ask for a break. You can say, "Hang on a sec, let's take a breath," "Let's slow things down," "Let's get a glass of water," or "Not right now."

If, however, you're sure this is a no, it's best to be clearer: "You know what? I'm not feeling this right now," "My body is a no," "This doesn't feel right," or "I'm kind of shut down right now."

I know it can be scary to assert yourself like this, but it is the best way to honor yourself, and the more you do it, the easier it will be. And by the way, any partner who doesn't respect your "no" isn't one you want to have!

If it is indeed a "Hell, yes," though, asking for and receiving consent doesn't have to ruin the moment. It can actually be really sexy to make asking for consent a part of seduction and foreplay. Instead of asking, "Is it okay to kiss you?" try, "I'm wondering what it would be like to kiss you." This is a very subtle distinction, but the former is simply asking for permission, while the latter is a bid for collaboration. Instead of feeling challenged to make a decision, it leads the other person to think, "Hmmm… I wonder if I would like that, as well…"

No matter how you ask, consent is a must, and it's best given before you're in the middle of things. Pregaming consent and talking about all of the hot stuff that you're going to do together does not have to be a mood killer. If you keep it flirty, it can actually increase desire and arousal. Laying out what's on the menu ahead of time allows you to freely play within the lines instead of worrying about whether your partner is going to cross a line and try something that's not your jam.

Remember that saying yes to sex or even to a particular sex act doesn't mean that you can't stop or pause and get clarity once it's started. As things progress, ask your partner how they're feeling and if what you're doing feels good to them. Likewise, tell your partner if you're not comfortable, if you want them to do something different, or if you want to take a break or slow down or stop. All of this is okay.

It's important to note that what you desire changes, and consent must be ongoing. Let's say that you and your partner agreed that they would tie you up, but once your wrists are bound, you start to feel a little panicky and stressed. You do not have to continue with this just because you agreed to it. Simply say, "Can we take a break for a minute?" And then explain how you're feeling to your partner. Anyone worth having sex with will be more than happy to recalibrate to make sure that what you are doing together is comfortable and pleasurable for both of you.

Along with mutual consent, it's important to make sure that you have clear boundaries when it comes to sex. It's not easy to articulate, enforce, or recognize boundaries. In fact, the entire concept of boundaries can take time to grasp, but the consensus in the sexual and mental health field is that learning to set and hold boundaries is an important part of healthy communication.

An easy way to think about this is that your boundaries are guidelines and limits, essentially specific instructions about how your partner should treat you. And your partner's boundaries are instructions on how they want to be treated.

It's difficult to know what to say to set a boundary on the spot, and when we do this we often end up being wishy-washy. We don't know what to say, so we don't say anything at all, or we say something unclear or half-hearted. It's a good idea to be clear about your boundaries ahead of time so this doesn't happen. The more you practice, the more comfortable you will get setting your own limits.

If you have a hard time setting boundaries, let's reprogram your thinking: boundaries help you relax. They establish trust. And, again, if someone does not respect your boundaries, that's a sexual partner you do not need to have.

Let's say that you want to consent to sex, but you have a boundary that using condoms is a must for you. Making this a clear boundary from the beginning is essential for your comfort, which will help you maximize your pleasure in the moment. If you've communicated this boundary and your partner disregards it or tries to talk you out of it, well, now you have some excellent information. Did they forget, or did they not hear you? Or do you need to reinforce the boundary? The more we stick to our boundaries, the more confidence we'll have in ourselves to be our own best advocates. We're also showing people how we need and expect to be treated.

Of course, it's just as important to respect and honor your partner's boundaries. If you bring up a sexual fantasy or make a request and they say no, thank them for being clear rather than trying to talk them into it. It's okay to get curious and ask them for more information about the boundary, such as its origin or what they're into, instead.

In a trusting and healthy relationship, once fantasy talk gets going, many partners will say no to things that are new to them or that they just don't understand. This is when you can get curious and find out what does turn your partner on. Sometimes when one partner says no to the other's fantasy, it can lead to a compromise where you both find something that works for you. Maybe your partner isn't into threesomes like you are, but you find out that they get turned on by talking about threesomes or watching threesome porn together. This is a beautiful collaboration where one partner is getting a need met and the other is learning more and is still able to please their partner while maintaining their boundary.

However, you don't ever want to pressure a partner into doing something they don't want to do. In fact, aggressively bypassing a partner's no can fall into the category of sexual coercion. Sexual coercion is wearing someone down, threatening, pressuring, lying, or manipulating someone into unwanted sexual activity. It is *very far* from pleasurable and, in certain power dynamics, it's even illegal. It's important to understand where that line is and not to cross it. That goes for your partner and for you, as well.

Keep in mind that when you start talking about sex for the first time, it can bring up a lot of our deeply buried insecurities and fears and even past traumas. When you and your partner take the time to reassure and support and really hear each other, it will help create a deeper connection, which almost always leads to hotter, better, and more satisfying sex.

Exercise: Sixty-Nine Questions

This is a fun and sexy game to play with your partner to open up the conversation about sex. To play, sit down facing one another. Stare deeply into each other's eyes. The first person to blink goes first. Start at the top of the list and then take turns answering each of the questions. Remember to practice active listening to get the most out of this. And of course, feel free to stop or pause the game to act out anything that turns you both on.

1. What part of your body do you find sexiest?
2. What part of your body do you want sexual compliments for?
3. Which celebrities turn you on?
4. What do you value most in a sexual relationship?

5. What are your top sexual turn-ons?
6. What are your sexual taboos?
7. When do you feel most sexually confident?
8. What are some of your sexual insecurities?
9. What do you find most beautiful or attractive about people?
10. What things or experiences are most sensual to you?
11. What haven't you tried sexually that you are curious about?
12. What sexual dreams do you remember?
13. What words turn you on?
14. What words turn you off?
15. What's your favorite way to refer to the vulva? The penis?
16. What foods turn you on?
17. How do you most like to be held?
18. What role-plays most intrigue you?
19. What did you learn from your parents about sex—the good, bad, and the ugly?
20. What's the most creative sex you've had?
21. What costumes or clothing get you hot?
22. What is your ideal foreplay?
23. How do you love to be kissed?
24. What is your fantasy sex vacation?
25. What specific touches turn you on the most?
26. What are your sexual pet peeves?
27. How are you best seduced?
28. What do you prefer: getting, giving, or mutuality?
29. What is sexual trust to you?
30. How rough or soft do you like it?
31. What do you need most to get in the mood for sex?
32. What gets you off the most: licking, penetration, hands, or...?
33. What are your sexual secrets?

34. How do you feel about domination and submission? Bondage?
35. What forbidden fantasies do you have?
36. What movies, music, or books turn you on?
37. What's the freest sexual thing you have ever done?
38. What is the most exotic place you have ever had sex?
39. What turns you on most when touching yourself?
40. Have you had any group sex experiences or fantasies?
41. What is the kinkiest sex you ever had?
42. What could you be more sexually open about?
43. When have you lied about sex?
44. What sexual rules have you broken?
45. Do you have any sexual regrets?
46. What freaks you out sexually?
47. What overwhelms you during sex?
48. Can you tell me about any sexual trauma I should be sensitive to?
49. How do you feel about getting drunk or high for sex?
50. What do you wish I understood about you sexually?
51. What heightens your arousal?
52. What kills your arousal?
53. What do you need most after sex?
54. When do you feel most emotionally close during sex?
55. What positions do you most enjoy?
56. What positions are not comfortable for you?
57. What embarrasses you sexually?
58. What grosses you out sexually?
59. What is a deal breaker for you in a sexual relationship?
60. What makes you relax most during sex?
61. What times of day are sexually prime for you?

62. What is your favorite sexual memory?
63. When you daydream about sex, what do you think about?
64. What do you love—or not love—about oral?
65. What do you love—or not love—about anal?
66. In the best of all possible worlds, how frequently would you want to have sex?
67. What is your preferred method of sexual protection?
68. What have you learned from your sexual mistakes?
69. If you could write a sexual autobiography, what would its title be?

Whether the conversation is about boundaries, consent, fantasies, or feedback, talking about sex isn't something that you can ever cross off your list and be done with. These conversations should be ongoing throughout your relationship so that you and your partner are intentionally building the sex life that you both desire. Using these tools will improve your relationship, help you collaborate, and will come in handy as we move on to more complex and nuanced sexual situations that are built on trust, intimacy, and top-notch communication.

5

Have Moregasms:

How to Maximize Your Orgasms

I have a confession to make. Over the last twenty years, I've gone from never having an orgasm and faking it whenever I had sex with a partner to being multi-orgasmic. My personal record is twenty-three orgasms in one night. I probably should have put this on the cover of the book!

We all covet orgasms. They are the ultimate source of pleasure, and they are good for our emotional and physical well-being. Every time we have an orgasm, our bodies release a powerful combination of hormones that improve our moods, reduce anxiety and stress, and boost our immune systems. Our bodies are built for pleasure!

Yet, orgasms remain mysterious and elusive. We rarely talk about them, even with our partners, and we often don't understand exactly how to have them or even how to tell if one has happened. Well, I say, let's stop leaving these healthy sources of intense pleasure to chance. It's time to take control and own your O.

Whatever your current relationship with orgasms is, you're going to find tips in this chapter to improve it. Maybe you've never had one, you've only had them alone but never with a partner, you think you have them too quickly, you think that it takes you too long, you can only have them one certain way, or you just want yours to be stronger and more powerful or more plentiful or just plain different. Rest assured that no matter what, this chapter has got you covered.

The Physiology of Orgasms

Let's start with the basics, since many of us don't know what an orgasm is exactly except for something that feels good. Orgasms are rhythmic contractions in the genitals and pelvic floor muscles following the height of sexual arousal. They are essentially the world's most pleasurable muscle spasms! For you to have an orgasm, a team effort is required between your nerve endings, blood flow, pelvic floor muscles, and that big sex organ in your head.

When your nerve endings register pleasurable sensations in your sex organs, they prompt your brain to send more blood to your genitals, heightening those nerve endings' sensitivity. Notice that I said pleasurable sensations. Your brain is in charge of interpreting the sensations in your sex organs and deciding whether or not you like them. If it decides that you don't, the orgasmic process will be over before it even starts.

If, however, your brain interprets that you do like what's happening, the orgasmic process begins. It starts with increased blood flow. No matter what kind of genitals you have, they will swell, grow in size, become erect and even lubricated as a result of this extra blood. If you have a penis, the paired corpus cavernosa and single corpus spongiosum are three spongy columns of erectile tissue that run through most of the shaft and fill with blood. Those engorged blood vessels create an erection. The penis also self-lubricates with a small amount of pre-ejaculate.

If you have a vulva, the clitoris grows and becomes erect, and the increased blood flow helps create vaginal lubrication, which is actually plasma that's been filtered from all that extra blood flow. If you have a vulva or a penis, your pelvic floor muscles also engorge with blood. If arousal is sustained, these muscles give way to the muscular contractions of orgasm.

Although some experts and researchers disagree with the idea that orgasm is a linear process, it is generally agreed that there are four stages of orgasm. Erotic desire, which starts in the brain, begins the process. In addition to increased blood flow to the genitals, nipples become erect, the breath quickens, and blood flushes to the surface of the skin, making it more sensitive.

Between arousal and orgasm is the plateau stage, when blood continues to flow, tissues remain erect and lubricated, and so on. Then there is a concentration of blood flow to the genitals, and it's orgasm time! Muscles contract, the brain releases a rush of hormones, and most penis owners (and some vulva owners) ejaculate.

Post-orgasm, there is a resolution stage when blood flows away from the genitals, your breathing slows and deepens, and hormones continue trickling in. Usually, a sense of calm and contentment settles in thanks to that powerful cocktail of hormones. They include:

Oxytocin: This is considered the "bonding hormone" because it promotes feelings of closeness and connection. Your brain releases oxytocin during skin-to-skin contact, such as when a mother breastfeeds her baby, when you cuddle with someone you love, and both during and after orgasm. It's also released when you hear the voice of a loved one! This explains why it feels so good to snuggle after sex and why so many people feel increased connection or even love for their partners after orgasming.

Estrogen: In addition to its other important roles, estrogen boosts collagen production, which helps explain why we often experience a glow after sex! As we discussed earlier, estrogen helps increase sex drive. This is one reason it's often true that the more sex you have, the more sex you want to have.

Endorphins: These are energy hormones that are also natural pain relievers. Orgasms can relieve menstrual cramps, back pain, and headaches.

Dopamine: As I discussed earlier, dopamine makes us feel good and motivates us to feel good again—another reason that sex can beget sex. Dopamine feeds on novelty, so trying new things in bed heightens the excitement and pleasure response. If your sexual routine feels stale, switching it up can promote dopamine production.

Serotonin: This happy hormone is a mood regulator that also promotes feelings of pride. When you have an orgasm and experience a release of serotonin, you feel happy and maybe even proud of yourself. Increased serotonin also lowers the stress hormone cortisol, reducing feelings of stress.

Prolactin: This hormone leads to milk production in lactating vulva owners, but we all release it during orgasm. It is associated with increased feelings of sleepiness, and prolactin levels can impact the refractory period (the time between having an orgasm and the ability to become aroused again). Interestingly, the release of prolactin during partnered orgasm is four hundred percent greater than it is during masturbation. This helps explain why some of us feel energized after orgasming during masturbation but fall asleep immediately after orgasming during partnered sex.

Now you know what all the fuss is about. Intense pleasure plus feelings of happiness, connection, and pride, less pain, reduced stress, and gleaming skin. Not bad at all. All orgasms create these wonderful effects, though there are many different kinds.

All Orgasms Are Created Equal

Orgasms are typically discussed in a binary and gendered way—the male orgasm and the female orgasm. But for vulva and penis owners alike, there are multiple ways to orgasm. Understanding each of them and how they happen in the body can help you experience them, help your partner experience them, or both.

First, some background on this topic. Orgasm science is understudied and ongoing. Just as I was writing this chapter, a new study came out that said the clitoris has ten thousand nerve endings, two thousand more than we previously believed! That old number came from studying a cow's clitoris, not even a human one. And the *New York Times* released an article with a headline stating that in terms of research, the clitoris is "completely ignored by pretty much everyone."

This has been the case for a long, long time. In 1905, Sigmund Freud theorized that clitoral orgasms were an "adolescent phenomenon," and that upon reaching puberty, vulva owners would graduate to vaginal orgasms, which happened during intercourse.

Of course, Freud had zero evidence for this theory. It wasn't until half a century later that sex researcher Alfred Kinsey became the first to criticize it after actually talking to vulva owners. Imagine that! He concluded that Freud's theory was wildly off base, inspiring a closer look at orgasms for vulva and penis owners alike.

But the impact of Freud's false theory was still huge and lasting. Even today, the way sex is depicted in mainstream media and porn is completely unrealistic. We often see a penis owner penetrate a vagina (with little to no foreplay or lube, by the way), and maybe thirty seconds later, the vulva owner is screaming and writhing in ecstasy.

This is off base and highly damaging, and has led to confusion, shame, and a persistent orgasm gap between vulva and penis owners, particularly vulva owners in heterosexual relationships. In heterosexual couples, ninety-five percent of penis owners report usually or always having an orgasm during a sexual experience with a partner. For vulva owners, that number was only sixty-five percent. For vulva owners in same-sex relationships, it was eighty-six percent. This makes sense, since vulva owners know firsthand how to bring a vulva to orgasm and how long it takes.

The one question people ask me more than pretty much any other comes from vulva owners and their partners. They want to know why the vulva owner can only have clitoral orgasms (mainly from oral or a vibrator) and doesn't orgasm during vaginal penetration. Penis owners fear that they're doing something wrong and not pleasing their partners, and vulva owners fear that they are somehow inadequate or broken if they don't experience orgasm during penetrative sex.

I get it. I used to feel this way, too. But then I learned the facts. In reality, up to eighty percent of vulva owners require external clitoral stimulation from a hand, mouth, or toy to have an orgasm. Only twenty percent have orgasms from vaginal penetration alone. Twenty percent!

If you're in the grand majority of vulva owners who don't orgasm from penetration alone, there is nothing whatsoever wrong with you. You are not broken or inadequate or "bad at sex." Your needs are legitimate and completely normal. If you want your partner to bring you to orgasm, ask for clitoral stimulation via a tongue or a hand or a toy. Far more often than not, the penis doesn't create an orgasm. Clitoral stimulation does.

In many cases, the ability of vulva owners to orgasm (or not) during penetration comes down to physiology, specifically the distance between the clitoris and the vaginal opening. Studies have suggested that people with a shorter distance experience orgasms more frequently during penetration. The location of their clitorises means that it's easier for them to receive more consistent stimulation during intercourse.

If you're a penis owner with a partner who has a vulva, the best thing you can do to help them orgasm is to let them know that their vulva is beautiful and that it would be your honor to dive in there no matter how long it takes to bring them to orgasm orally or however they prefer.

On average, during partnered sex, it takes penis owners about five minutes to orgasm while it takes vulva owners eighteen minutes or more with a partner. While the exact percentages might vary by studies, it's important to note that penis owners typically have an orgasm a lot quicker, and more frequently, than vulva owners. This leads many vulva owners to feel insecure or guilty about how hard their partner is "working." If their partners don't know the facts, it can make them feel like they're doing something wrong. These feelings are all pleasure thieves!

The more you relax, get rid of any and all expectations, and focus on the sensations in your body, the more pleasure you will be able to give and receive. I can't tell you how many times I found myself staring at the clock when a guy was going down on me, thinking it was taking too long. *It's already been fifteen minutes, I better wrap this up!* This is no away to orgasm. The more nonsexy thoughts we're having, the less likely we are to orgasm—or have any pleasure, for that matter.

Bottom line—while having an orgasm is not the entire point of sex, all orgasms are wonderful and healthy and special. No one type is "better" or more advanced than another. There is no orgasm hierarchy! But we do now know that there are several different types of orgasm. They are:

Penile Orgasm

This is the classic and most common type of orgasm for penis owners. It results primarily from stimulation of the head, shaft, frenulum, and foreskin of the penis (if the foreskin is present). Right before orgasm, seminal fluid, which helps escort semen out of the body, builds up at the base of the penis. It is then pushed out of the urethra through contractions of the pelvic floor and penile muscles, creating an orgasm and ejaculation.

Penis Anatomy

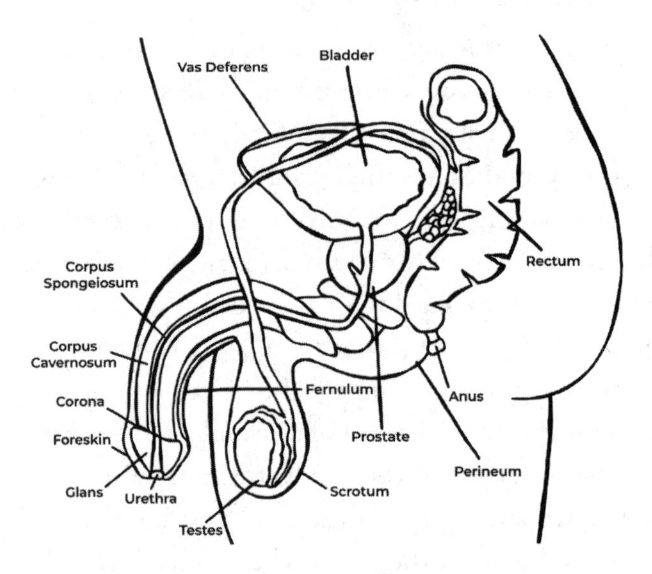

Penis Anatomy

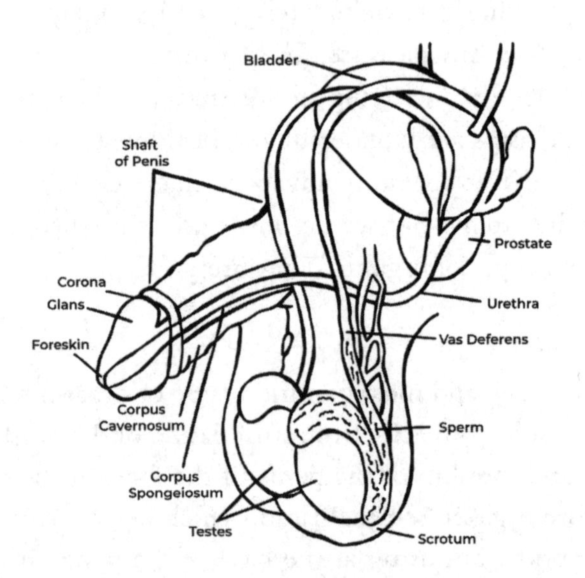

Prostate Orgasm

Accessible only through the anus and only in bodies with penises, the prostate is located just below the bladder. When stimulated through anal play, the prostate can produce an internal orgasm for penis owners. Interestingly, this type of orgasm can occur with or without an erection.

Dry Orgasm

Penis owners can have an orgasm without ejaculating—hence the term *dry*. The most common reason an orgasm is "dry" is that the penis owner has already had an orgasm and the well has run…well, dry, but they can still get erect and experience the muscle contractions of orgasm. After a break, the body will produce enough semen to ejaculate again.

Dry orgasms can also occur when semen isn't expelled from the tip of the penis and instead flows backward into the bladder. This isn't a cause for concern. That semen will likely just leave the body the next time the person urinates.

Semen retention is the process of learning to intentionally have a dry orgasm. This has become a bit of a trend lately, but it has actually been around for over five thousand years. According to the tantric sex tradition, retaining semen enhances the life force energy. More practically speaking, it might help penis owners maintain an erection after orgasm to last longer before ejaculation, as well as lead to multiple orgasms for penis owners. Research has shown it can also improve sperm motility and potentially increase testosterone levels.

A good time to try having a dry orgasm is after you've already ejaculated—ideally more than once. If the well is dry, so to speak, and you continue stimulating yourself sexually, it's more likely that you'll orgasm without ejaculating. Another way to practice semen retention is to work on edging. This will help you become aware of when you are about to ejaculate and retain it while still experiencing an orgasm.

Coregasm

Believe it or not, this is an orgasm that happens while you're doing a core exercise. It can definitely make your workout a lot more exciting! When you engage your muscles to stabilize your core, you may also contract the pelvic floor muscles, leading to an orgasm. Some penis owners ejaculate during a coregasm, while others don't.

For vulva owners, a coregasm feels similar to a deep vaginal orgasm with most sensation in the lower abdominals, inner thighs, or pelvis. I'll never forget the first time I had one of these on the thigh abductor machine at the gym!

Nipple-gasm

In vulva owners, nipple stimulation can activate the same region of the brain as the clitoris and the vagina: the genital sensory cortex. Because nipples are filled with nerve endings, continuous play may lead to an orgasm, especially in people who are more sensitive. Even if nipple play doesn't end in an orgasm, it can enhance arousal all over your body. Keep in mind that everyone's nipples are different—some people have little to no sensitivity, while others feel so sensitive they might prefer to skip nipple play entirely.

Blended Orgasm

When more than one erogenous zone is stimulated at the same time, it can lead to a blended orgasm. For example, this could be from simultaneous penile and prostate orgasm or a simultaneous clitoral and vaginal for a vulva owner. For vulva owners, this is more likely to happen when external clitoral stimulation is combined with another erogenous zone. For many, this makes it easier to experience a blended orgasm. Having sex toys on hand can help make this a reality.

Clitoral Orgasm

While the clitoris is the famous pleasure button that's visible outside of the body, it's actually a much larger organ than originally thought. Think of it like an iceberg: the top/the tip of it is visible, but most of it is actually below the surface. The part of the clitoris that we can see—the glans—is connected to clitoral legs called crura and clitoral bulbs called the vestibular bulbs that reach up *inside* the body. The crura form a V-shaped wishbone-like structure that surrounds your vaginal canal and urethra. This structure is packed with hypersensitive nerve endings, prompting an orgasm when the clitoris itself is stimulated. And because it is both an external and internal organ, it's possible to stimulate it from the outside *and* the inside of the vagina.

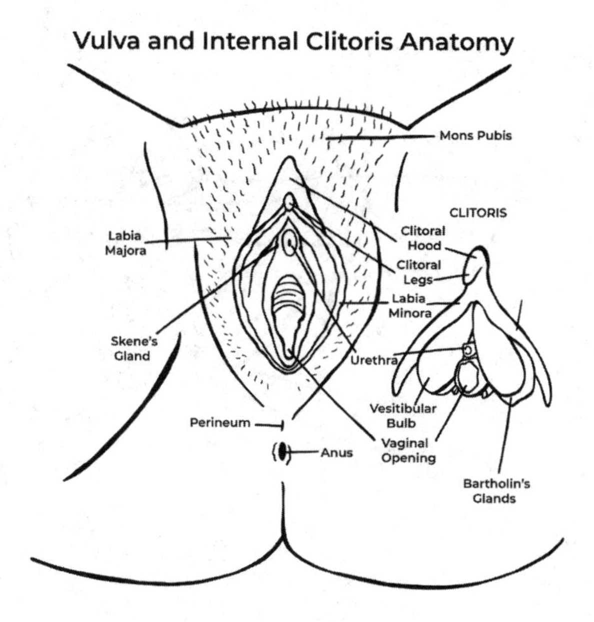

Cervical Orgasm

Also called the C-spot, the cervix is sensitive and has the potential to create a deep internal orgasm since it is located high inside the vaginal canal. Some vulva owners describe this as more of a full-body orgasm, with sensations beginning in the cervix and spreading out through the entire abdomen. However, many people find it uncomfortable or even painful to have their cervixes stimulated, and if that's you, you're not alone.

G-Area Orgasm

Located about two inches up the vaginal wall, the G-area sits just below your Skene's glands, which serve a similar function as the prostate gland in a penis owner. They produce the fluid responsible for female ejaculation. This is why G-area stimulation is necessary for female ejaculation.

Vagina Anatomy and Reproductive Organs

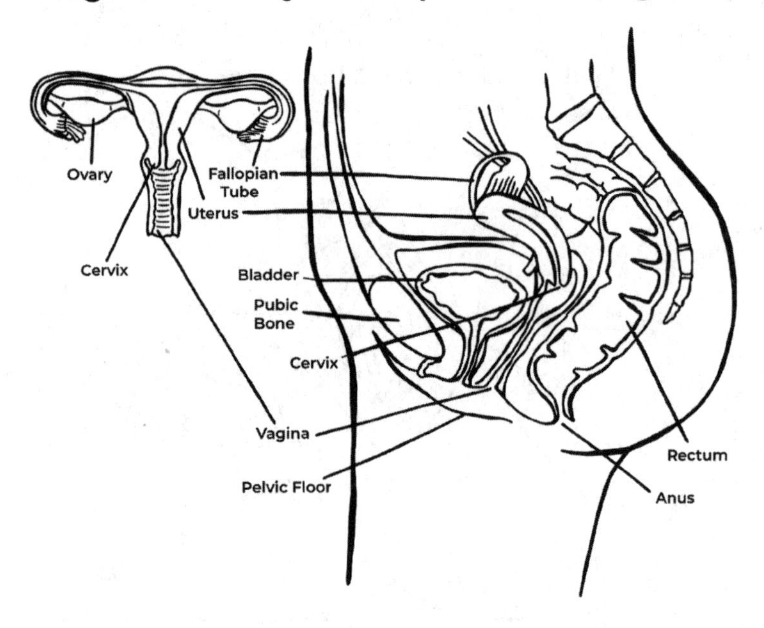

A-Spot Orgasm

In between the G-area and your cervix, there's also the A-spot (referring to the anterior fornix) and U-spot (referring to the urethra). All of these "spots" simply describe various locations on the interior walls of the vaginal canal. Their nerve endings can be stimulated to help prompt orgasm.

The G-Area Is Not a Myth—And Neither Is Squirting

Vagina Pleasure Points

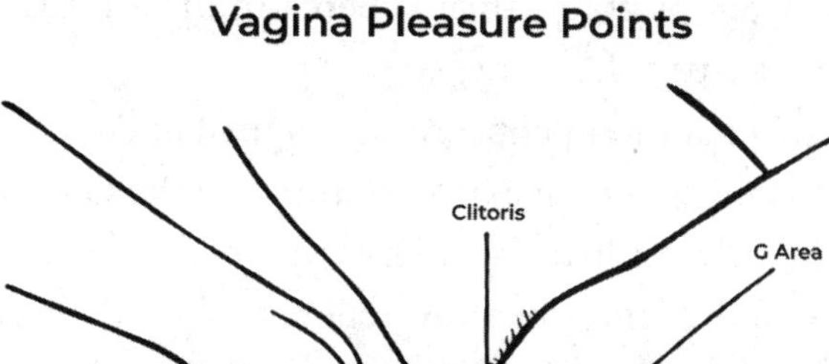

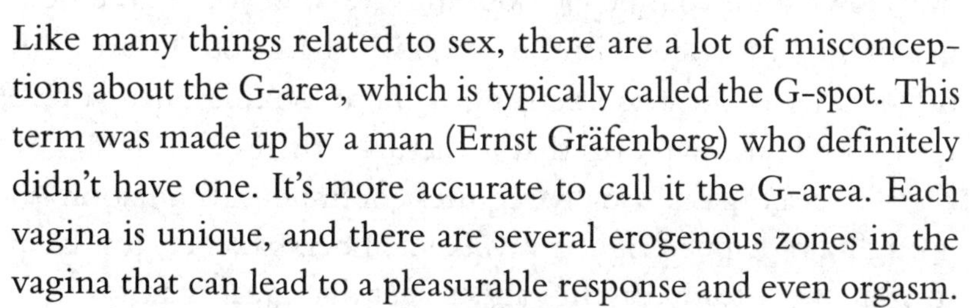

Like many things related to sex, there are a lot of misconceptions about the G-area, which is typically called the G-spot. This term was made up by a man (Ernst Gräfenberg) who definitely didn't have one. It's more accurate to call it the G-area. Each vagina is unique, and there are several erogenous zones in the vagina that can lead to a pleasurable response and even orgasm.

In general, the G-area is located about two inches inside of the vagina, perched on the front vaginal wall. Although its exact size and location may vary from vagina to vagina, you can most commonly locate it by feeling its ridged texture. It feels sort of like a walnut, although not everyone has this ridged texture. When a vulva owner becomes aroused, this lump of tissue swells and becomes more prominent and sensitive to the touch.

There is also the O-spot, a spongy tissue on the back wall of the vagina, and the A-zone, which is five or six inches deep inside an aroused vagina alongside the cervix, under the belly button. These areas, plus the nerves in your cervix, create a collection of erogenous zones that, when stimulated, can lead to orgasm for many people.

Contrary to what most people think, vaginal intercourse with a penis is not the most effective way to stimulate the G-area. I recommend that vulva owners begin by exploring solo. Once they know the lay of the land, they can report back to their partners.

To find the G-area, start with your palm facing up, and insert one or two fingers into your vagina. Gently stroke around the top of the vaginal wall. When you find the slightly ridged or protruding area, you might gasp a little or react with surprise. That means you're on the right track. Once you've located the area, stroke it with your index and middle finger using a come-hither motion. Play around with different amounts of pressure until you find what works, and then stick with it.

You can also find the G-area visually. Use a hand mirror to look at your vulva and use your fingers to part your labia. Now bear down with your pelvic floor muscles. Can you see the flesh expanding into view with ridges on it? That's your G-area. It's often easier to locate something without looking once you've seen with your own eyes that it's actually there.

A G-area orgasm usually requires continuous stimulation, so it might not happen right away. Remember, patience. Just keep stroking in a steady rhythm and accept that great orgasms usually take time. If your fingers aren't dexterous enough or they get tired, you can always bring a sex toy into play.

For some vulva owners, having a G-area orgasm is easier when you bring clitoral stimulation into the mix. This is why I recommend starting your G-area exploration with a clitoral orgasm. This will bring blood flow to the G-area, making it easier for you to have another orgasm. If it feels good, continue stimulating the clitoris as you explore your G-area.

When you start having G-area orgasms, you may experience

something else that is a source of major mystery and curiosity—squirting, aka female ejaculation.

It turns out that most vulva owners can learn to ejaculate, even if they never have. One study of vulva owners all over the world showed that sixty-nine percent of them were able to shoot fluid from the urethra when experiencing sexual pleasure. Using an ultrasound machine, they witnessed once-empty bladders slowly fill with fluid during solo sex and expel it during orgasm. Though it came from the bladder, the fluid wasn't urine. It's produced by the Skene's glands, often called the female prostate because it shares the same structure as the prostate in bodies with penises.

Most vulva owners have two Skene's glands, one on each side of the urethra. Their main job is to secrete fluid into the urethra to keep it lubricated. When the G-area is stimulated in just the right way for enough time, the Skene's glands can secrete fluid into the urethra that can expel out during orgasmic muscle contractions.

On average, the volume of female ejaculate is two ounces of either clear or milky white fluid that's basically made of the same materials as semen, minus the sperm. Many people are concerned about whether the fluid expelled is urine. Some urine might be expelled, but remember that sex is messy, and throwing a towel down is an easy fix. It can trickle or shoot out with some force. Before ejaculating, it feels similar to having to pee, but when the fluid squirts out, it's a pleasurable surprise and a thrilling release. It's nothing to be embarrassed about or ashamed of. The vast majority of squirters find that their special skill enriches their sex lives, and most of the time, their partners are into it.

Since the G-area needs to be stimulated in order to ejaculate, start by following the steps above—enjoy a clitoral orgasm, back off, stay aroused, and then find the G-area. When you're stimulating the G-area, remember to go slow. The nerves that you're stimulating are deep and internal. This requires patience. You're building up tension for an orgasmic release, and it takes time to engorge the erectile tissue of your G-area. Stroke with a slow, steady rhythm.

If you feel that sensation of needing to pee, you're on the right track. But don't be horrified if you do end up peeing a little. It will take a little time for your brain to pick up on the subtle distinction between impending ejaculation and actually needing to urinate. Until then, put a towel down and roll with it. Sex is messy. We're human animals, and a little pee never hurt anyone.

Once you feel that "I have to pee" sensation, try to relax the muscles in the pelvic floor. Breathe deeply, and take everything out of your vagina that you've got in there—whether it's a toy, a penis, or fingers. Most vulva owners can't ejaculate with anything inside of their vaginas.

Now, as you feel the orgasmic contractions begin, bear down with your belly and pelvic floor muscles. This enables a clear pathway for the ejaculate to come out. I want to make it clear that vulvas can ejaculate with or without orgasm. For many vulva owners, it's an intense release, but not one that necessarily ends in a mind-blowing orgasm.

Squirting has become a popular "sex goal" over the past twenty years, thanks to porn. But not every vulva owner wants or is able to experience ejaculation. Worry not! There are plenty of other ways of finding immense pleasure. This is just one option on a very long and exciting menu.

Don't Stop at Just One

While penis owners may appear to have an advantage in terms of their ability to orgasm more quickly, vulva owners have an advantage when it comes to experiencing that pleasure in multiples. When we talk about multiple orgasms, we can mean having more than one orgasm during the same sex session or arousal state, say an hour apart, or we can mean having more than one orgasm in a row, with one rolling right into the next with only twenty or thirty seconds in between.

Vulva owners have the advantage here because they have a shorter refractory time. Penis owners need more time after orgasm before they can get aroused (and orgasm) again. This could be a matter of minutes or a matter of hours.

As you get older, you might require between twelve and twenty-four hours before you're ready to go again. This is totally normal, but if you're looking to shorten your refractory period, exercise helps. Cardiovascular health is directly linked to blood flow, which you need for erection and orgasm.

I believe that all vulva owners can learn to have multiple orgasms, but it usually takes some time and effort. Try not to put pressure on yourself (or your partner) or feel "less than" if you don't succeed. The first thing you need is patience. Stick with it, and eventually you'll be amazed at how much pleasure your body can deliver.

As a first step to experiencing multiple orgasms, I recommend exploring your body on your own with your favorite masturbation techniques. Like I said, it's often easier to have an internal orgasm (like a G-area orgasm) after a clitoral one because the genitals are already engorged. So, it's key to prioritize clitoral stimulation with a toy (or oral sex if you're with a partner) before you aim for additional Os.

After you experience your first orgasm, you might feel sensitive and need to pull back from direct stimulation of the clitoris. This is a great time to turn your focus to other sensitive areas of your body, like the nipples, to maintain your arousal. This is also a good time to remember to breathe. One trick in achieving multiple orgasms is to stay connected to your body mentally and physically after the first orgasm. Slow down and focus on each inhale and exhale. Breathing will relax your body and expand your pleasure potential.

Deep breaths also flood your body with oxygen so your nervous system can do its job, increasing the amount of pleasure that your brain can process. If you get overwhelmed or frustrated and shorten your breath, you'll likely shut down your body from pleasure. I visualize the breath going straight into my pelvis, filling the clitoris itself.

Also, don't be afraid to get loud. Making any kind of vibrating sound like moaning or humming stimulates the vagus nerve that runs down either side of your neck and winds all the way down to the cervix. If you moan when having an orgasm, it keeps you in a relaxed, parasympathetic nervous system state, which allows you to feel more sensation.

For the second orgasm, crank down the vibe power level, and tease yourself a little bit. Use it to lightly trace over your nipples, your pelvic mound, and all over your body to find out what other areas heighten your arousal. When you feel that you're ready, try using a toy that's designed for internal (G-area) stimulation.

If you want to return to the hot spot, try different techniques like indirect touches, cupping, or rubbing the area around the clitoris. Vary the position, pressure, and speed of your stroke to introduce new sensations. Then slowly crank up the power to carry you over the plateau and into orgasm oblivion.

Orgasm Enhancers

While all orgasms are wonderful, some are stronger than others with more pleasurable sensations, and there are ways to make them even more powerful. Here are a few tricks to make yours as potent as possible.

Edging

Edging is the practice of building up to orgasms by repeatedly getting to the brink and then backing off so that the eventual release is more controlled and even more pleasurable. This is a technique that serves a dual purpose. It can help make your orgasms more powerful no matter what genitals you have. Penis owners can also use this technique to control premature ejaculation.

Technically, the term premature ejaculation refers to a relatively rare medical condition in which a penis owner consistently ejaculates within one minute of penetration, and feels that they have no control over it. But at some point, one in three penises ejaculates before their owner wants it to. The causes can be medical or psychological, and edging can be highly effective in helping to prevent it.

For vulva owners, edging is more about building intensity. I get that many vulva owners feel like they're climbing Mount Everest just to have an orgasm. Why would you want to stop it? But when you edge, you don't slide all the way back down, and eventually climb higher and higher.

The first step is to become familiar with the "edging scale." On a scale of one to ten, one is feeling nothing and ten is having an orgasm. To practice edging, you'll want to work your way up to a seven or eight once or twice before allowing yourself to get to a ten.

It's great to start practicing edging during solo sex. I recommend using your hands at first. The process of edging is all about attuning to your body's signals. Vibrators are so appealing because their intensity gets you to orgasm quickly, but edging is about building slowly before coming back down. Of course, if you really prefer a vibrator, go for it. Try experimenting with different speeds and pulse patterns to mix it up.

As you go, pay attention to the signs in your body that you are approaching orgasm. Is your breath changing? Which body parts are tensing up? How is your heart rate changing? Make a note of the subtle shifts, and over time you'll be able to fine-tune your approach. Even if you don't succeed at first, you'll still have an orgasm as a consolation prize! You'll also gain self-awareness around what it takes to get you to the point of no return.

If you're edging with a partner, talk to them about your intentions and stay connected throughout, using verbal and non-verbal cues. Maybe come up with a code word that means you're getting close and want to back off. Then start again slowly with kissing, mutual masturbation, oral teasing, or whatever form of foreplay you like. Remember to breathe!

Steadily increase the intensity with more touching, penetration, or toys until you reach that number seven or eight, and then pause or reduce stimulation. Repeat this process one or two more times until you decide to go for that big finish. Each time, you can try to let yourself get closer and closer. For example, go for a seven during your first round and then an eight and then a nine... If you can't stop in time and orgasm before you'd like, who cares?

Toys

Experimenting with sex toys is a great way to enhance your orgasms. If you're looking for a toy to enhance your solo sex, refer back to Chapter 3. Here, I'll focus on the best toys for increased and varied orgasms during partnered sex.

Many partners are nervous about using toys together for the first time. Some even think that if they need a toy, they're failing their partner as a lover. The truth is that sex toys are built to do things that our bodies literally cannot do, like pulse and vibrate and perfectly reach nooks and crannies deep inside our bodies. They are simply effective tools to stimulate nerve endings that are difficult to access, and they can add sensations that make partnered sex varied and interesting. If you or your partner is nervous or intimidated or overwhelmed, I recommend going shopping for a new toy together to build comfort, anticipation, and excitement.

I wish I could wave my magic wand (one of my all-time most beloved vibrators) and erase all the stigma, worries, and shame around what using a vibrator means. Penis owners often worry that a vibrator is going to replace them, while vulva owners worry that they'll get addicted to their vibrators or that it's somehow wrong to use one...like we're cheating on an orgasm test and our orgasm doesn't count if it comes from a vibrator. Nothing could be further from the truth. Think about it this way—going into a sexual experience, penis owners pretty much always know that they're going to orgasm, while vulva owners often worry that they won't. Using vibrators is a way of removing those worries. They're an additive, not a replacement.

Vibrators can be enhancements for penis owners, too. I highly recommend trying a vibrating penis ring. Regular penis rings (or cock rings) are used to keep blood trapped in the penis to maintain engorgement. Vibrating penis rings have the secondary benefit of stimulating the nerve endings in the perineum, which also hardens when the penis gets erect. The perineum connects to the pudendal nerve, and it is also sensitive. For penis owners who have no trouble getting erect but have a harder time crossing the finish line, vibrating penis rings can be miracle workers. Look for a toy with a range of gentle vibrations.

There are also vibrating penis rings that are designed to provide clitoral stimulation during penetration. For many vulva owners, this can be the golden ticket to finally orgasming during penetrative sex, since, I repeat, eighty percent of us don't orgasm from penetration alone.

Another option is to use a bullet vibrator or other vibe with a flexible shape that you can mold as you like on the clitoris during sex. For example, try a position where you and your partner are facing away from each other, such as spooning or doggy style. If your partner has a penis, they can penetrate you from behind while they (or you) use the vibrator to stimulate your clitoris.

These days, there are also plenty of hands-free, wearable vibrators that are designed to stimulate two partners simultaneously during penetrative sex. For penis-in-vulva penetration, look for toys that tuck into the labia. Once in place, they stimulate the clitoris and the base of the penis. There are also insertable toys that stimulate the clitoris and the G-area as well as the shaft of the penis as it thrusts, and double-ended dildos with two heads for double penetration.

It might take you some time to get the hang of using toys and to build them into your routine. It might even feel awkward at first. That's okay! There are three things that will help here more than anything: an open mind, open communication with your partner, and of course, an open bottle of lube.

Kegels

The pelvic floor is like a hammock that supports some very important organs like your uterus, bladder, and bowels—it's not only an important player in childbirth, but it also impacts your sexual health. Because orgasms stem from the pelvic floor muscles, the stronger those muscles are, the more powerful your orgasm is going to be. When your pelvic floor is strong and toned, you'll have more muscle fibers available to stimulate your genital nerve endings before and during orgasm. Kegel exercises are simply a workout for your pelvic floor muscles.

Many of us have heard about how important it is for vulva owners to do Kegel exercises, but they're essential for penis owners, too. For penis owners, toning the pelvic floor often results in more projectile-like ejaculations. For vulva owners, toning the pelvic floor often results in deeper, more internal orgasms.

Regardless of what genitals you have, to give your pelvic floor a workout, empty your bladder first, and then sit or lie down comfortably. Take a few deep breaths to encourage your blood to flow throughout your body. Now squeeze your muscles as if you are trying to stop the flow of urine. Hold the muscles tight for three to five seconds and then release. Wait three to five seconds, and then squeeze them again.

Repeat this ten times, three times a day—once in the morning, once in the afternoon, and once at night. The whole process should only take a minute or two, and the results can be really pleasurable and profound. Please keep in mind that Kegels are not a one-size-fits-all cure-all, and there are conditions that can arise from having too tight of a pelvic floor. Vaginismus involves involuntary contractions of the pelvic floor that can make penetration painful. It is treatable through pelvic floor physical therapy, so don't despair. But if you have a vulva and it hurts when you insert a finger, toy, or penis, hold off on doing your Kegels for now and see a physical therapist who specializes in pelvic floor rehabilitation.

If Kegels are right for you, there is also a variety of tools available to help with them, ranging from Kegel weights that are placed in the vagina to high-tech stimulation devices that use electrical currents to activate your pelvic floor. Many vulva owners attempt to do Kegels but don't know how to do them correctly. I highly recommend pelvic floor muscle strengtheners that do the work of Kegels for you.

Breathe Your Way to Orgasm

It is possible to orgasm without any direct stimulation (touching) simply through the power of the breath. This can be tricky to master, but on the bright side, practicing will also strengthen your pelvic floor muscles and help you become more embodied. The result is often a more powerful orgasm regardless of how you get there.

To start, take three deep breaths into your belly and exhale slowly. Next, do the same thing, but this time, bring your awareness to your genitals. How do they feel? Come up with an adjective to describe it. Are they numb or tingly or warm or something else?

Continue taking slow, deep breaths with your eyes closed, imaging the breath traveling down through your throat to your chest, belly, and genitals. After a few rounds, bring your awareness to your pelvic floor muscles. As you inhale, squeeze those muscles as if you're stopping the flow of urine. Hold your breath for a second while holding them tight and then exhale slowly. Try to release your muscles at the same time that you release your breath. Practice syncing up your Kegels with your breath. As you inhale, squeeze your muscles, and as you exhale, release.

Once you've gotten this rhythm down, slow your breath even more, and inhale as if you're sucking in air through a straw while constricting those pelvic floor muscles. Then slowly release the air as if you're exhaling through a straw. Don't fully release the muscles until you release all of the air.

If you practice this enough, you might find that you're able to create an orgasm through the synchronicity of your breath and pelvic floor contractions. Even if you don't, you've exercised your pelvic floor, shifted your nervous system into a calm, parasympathetic state, and gotten in touch with your body.

O Blockers

If you're reading all of this feeling frustrated because you've never orgasmed, it's very likely that you are pre-orgasmic, meaning you are capable of having an orgasm but haven't had one yet, rather than anorgasmic, meaning you are truly unable to have one. Only about ten percent of vulva owners suffer from anorgasmia. This diagnosable condition is caused by physical issues like neurological disease, aging, addiction, and emotional and psychological factors like PTSD, severe body image issues, and deep shame.

If you try all of the tips in this chapter and still aren't able to have an orgasm and never have, consider talking to a doctor who specializes in sexual health about whether or not you may have anorgasmia. But assuming that you are pre-orgasmic, which is much more common, my biggest piece of advice is to commit to a solo sex practice. This will help train your neural pathways to experience pleasure.

Oh, and lube. Always lube. According to research from the

Kinsey Institute, vulva owners are eighty percent more likely to orgasm when they use lube. I hope that one day there will be a bottle of lube on every nightstand.

If you've had orgasms in the past but can't seem to get over the hump (so to speak) now, it's important to know that certain lifestyle factors reduce sexual sensitivity and blood flow. Drinking excess alcohol, eating foods that don't make you feel good, smoking, lack of exercise, and taking certain medications can all inhibit orgasms.

As we discussed earlier, understanding how your lifestyle and overall health is affecting your orgasm is an important part of your Sex IQ. If you're missing your O, consider making small changes like eating better and exercising, drinking less alcohol before sex, cutting down on smoking, and looking into your medications' potential side effects. Also make sure to go to the doctor for regular checkups and talk to them about this.

Sometimes, there is a more complex medical issue at play. Hormonal changes, such as decreased estrogen or testosterone, can inhibit orgasm. With age, we naturally start to experience fewer orgasms, and this is usually due to those reduced levels of sex hormones. Talk to your doctor and think about seeing a hormone specialist who may be able to support you with hormone replacement therapy (if appropriate).

Our mental health also plays a huge role in our ability to orgasm. Remember, your brain is your biggest sex organ. I'll keep repeating this until it sinks in—if you're having a lot of thoughts before, during, or after sex that don't serve you, they will have a direct impact on your ability to orgasm. When your brain is distracted, worried, anxious, or depressed, it can keep you from your O. The good news is that once you know that your brain is the problem, you can learn to navigate it. Your brain is very malleable and you can rewire it to experience more pleasure.

As we discussed, pleasure is presence. We can't get fully

aroused and orgasm if our brains are distracted by thoughts of tomorrow's big meeting, worries about how we look, or concerns about our "performance" in bed. Negative self-talk or feelings of guilt, fear, or shame can steal your orgasm here by telling your brain that something is wrong. Your brain will interpret this message as meaning that you don't like the sensations you're feeling and halt the arousal process.

Basically, anything that tells your brain that something is wrong will keep your body focused on survival instead of prioritizing pleasure. This is why problems and conflict in our relationships can also keep us from orgasming. If we don't feel completely safe and comfortable with our partners, we won't be able to let go and O.

Ironically, one common worry that can keep us from orgasming is about whether or not we're going to be able to orgasm! This is why I always say that orgasms are not the goal of sex. They're great, but it's counterproductive to put pressure on yourself (or your partner) to have one. Remember, in order to orgasm you have to be fully present in the moment, not stressed about whether or not you will have an orgasm or if you're getting close. The more you "try" to have an orgasm, the less likely you are to do so.

It's not necessary to have an orgasm in order to experience profound pleasure during partnered sex. There are so many other sensual delights to be had, and by being close and vulnerable and giving your partner pleasure, it's possible to be fully satisfied by the experience without having an orgasm yourself.

Orgasm might be the peak, but it's not the pleasure mountain. Don't miss out on the joy of climbing that mountain by worrying about peaking. If you focus on what you're feeling in the moment instead, you won't be derailed by negative thoughts, and you'll be more open to the sensations that will carry you over the mountain into the freefall of orgasm.

Exercise—Watch Yourself

One thing that can block us from the pleasure of orgasm is feeling self-conscious about how we look, sound, or act when we're in the throes of pleasure. I understand that it can be scary to lose control, especially in front of another person. It can make you feel very exposed and vulnerable.

When you're worried about your orgasm face or the sounds you make during orgasm and it keeps you from being fully present, you're robbing yourself of one of life's greatest pleasures. Plus, I have never in my life heard someone say that they didn't want to have sex with their partner again because they made a weird face or sound during orgasm. For most people, seeing their partner fully let go like that is actually a turn-on.

If you're still feeling unsure, exposure therapy can help. The website Beautiful Agony shows videos of people's faces as they orgasm—just the face. Seeing how beautiful and erotic these videos are will hopefully convince you that your own orgasm is incredibly sexy, too.

Why not find out for sure? Set up a mirror near your bed or couch and masturbate. When the big moment comes, open your eyes and watch yourself. This is a powerful way of gaining self-knowledge and self-acceptance, boosting your Sex IQ. Besides finally knowing what you look like as you orgasm, you'll gain a visual representation of what has always been just a feeling. This can be an added source of pleasure the next time you feel the pleasure of orgasm.

Whether you use the tools in this chapter to have your first orgasm ever, your first orgasm with a partner, multiple orgasms, a different kind of orgasm, or extra powerful orgasms, you're on your way to experiencing more and more pleasure. And you're learning new things about your body, which is powerful.

I'll say it one more time—orgasms are wonderful, but they're not the goal. Absorb this information, play around with it, and then let it go and allow yourself to enjoy yourself in every sexual scenario with no pressure and no goal other than to give and receive pleasure. Orgasms are the icing on the cake, but pleasure, in all its forms, is the cake itself.

6

Get Down with Going Down:

How to Give and Receive Embodied Oral Sex

In my early thirties, I was dating a guy who I'll call Jack. Early on in our relationship, he went down on me about as often as I went down on him, which was pretty damn often. But after a few months, he cut back to only about once a month, and then it was once every couple of months. Eventually, he just stopped doing it at all.

By then, I had learned enough about my own sexuality to know that oral is a primary source of my arousal and pleasure. This is the case with most vulva owners. I also knew how important it was for our relationship to have healthy communication about our sex life. So, I followed my own advice. Jack and I were in Malibu for a romantic weekend together. I knew he'd be relaxed and hoped he'd be receptive to having an open conversation about our sex life.

We sat down to dinner, and over a glass of wine I said, "Jack, I have a question for you. What do you think about our sex life?"

He seemed surprised by the question. "Oh my God, it's amazing," he said. "Things are great. What about you?"

"Well," I said carefully, "you know that I love oral sex. It feels so good when you go down on me. I've noticed that it hasn't happened in a long time, and I'm curious about why. Is it that you don't like it, or are you not sure how to do it so that I'll like it?"

I'd spoken to enough penis owners by then to know that many of them loved giving oral sex. If they shied away from it, it was usually because they weren't sure that they were doing it right and were too afraid to ask. "If you're not sure about what I want," I added a bit flirtatiously, "I'd be happy to teach you."

"It's not that," Jack said. "It's just not my thing."

The conversation ended there. We had our dinner and drank our wine. There wasn't much else to say on the topic. I had made my feelings clear, and he'd given me an honest answer. It was obvious to me that Jack wasn't going to come around on this. Giving oral "wasn't his thing." He had decided that no matter how much I wanted it, he wasn't going to do it.

Part of me wished I had asked sooner, but that night I realized that I had been putting off the conversation because I didn't want to deal with the consequences of not getting the answer I wanted. It would have been a much easier problem to solve if he'd just been feeling insecure about how to please me.

I told myself that at least now I had the information I needed, and I could use that information to make the decision that was best for me. I could sacrifice one of my main sources of sexual pleasure and continue in this relationship, or I could end it and find someone who loved giving me the kind of pleasure I wanted.

Twenty-five-year-old Emily would have stayed in that relationship for at least another year, convincing herself that he was good enough, at least on paper, and questioning if sex was really that important. I'd put off the inevitable until I met someone else or just couldn't take the lack of pleasure any longer.

But it had taken me a long time to learn to prioritize my pleasure, and I wasn't going to go backward. Plus, if Jack wasn't interested in collaborating with me on this, I knew that didn't bode well for our relationship in general.

I decided that if giving oral wasn't his thing, then Jack wasn't my thing.

The Truth About Oral Sex

Does it sound to you like I was being selfish or maybe putting too great of an emphasis on sex? Well, how would you feel about a penis owner who broke up with a partner because they wouldn't give blow jobs? Would that be any different? Regardless of our genitals, I wish we all learned to prioritize our own pleasure, along with our partner's.

Rather than selfishness, I see it as a healthy sense of entitlement. It wasn't just that I missed the sensations and orgasms that I received through oral (though I did). I also missed the eroticism that comes with it—a feeling of total acceptance from my partner and the complete surrender that comes with this particular sex act.

Giving and receiving oral sex is an integral part of being sexually healthy and of being a good lover, period. It's incredibly intimate to expose yourself fully to a partner who wants to give you pleasure. Plus, it's affirming, as it communicates "I want all of you." This can make you feel worthy, desired, and incredibly turned on.

It's not just me who thinks that oral sex is important. Michigan State University analyzed data from 884 heterosexual couples about their general happiness, self-reported mental health, and sexual practices. They found that both giving and receiving oral sex was positively correlated with feelings of happiness. In fact, people got the biggest bump in happiness from giving rather than receiving. The researchers concluded that oral sex might very well be the key to maintaining a happy, satisfying relationship over time. I say we follow the science on that one.

And yet, so many people still have issues with both giving and receiving oral sex. A quarter of Americans say that oral sex isn't fun, and another quarter say that oral sex makes them feel self-conscious. I long for this to change, but there is a good reason for it, or at least an understandable one.

First of all, oral sex was considered taboo until fairly recently. Believe it or not, some states still have laws banning oral sex on the books. Don't worry, a 2003 Supreme Court ruling declared these laws unconstitutional and therefore unenforceable. You are not going to get arrested for going down on your partner, but the taboo aspect of this sex act still lingers.

In recent years, blow jobs have gotten good PR and have become expected in most relationships that include at least one penis owner. But the way they've been portrayed in the media has inflated their importance in an unhealthy way that ties them to the giver's self-worth. Think about all those headlines that say things like "Learn how to give the best blow job, and any man will fall in love with you!" Does this mean that you're not lovable if you don't give the "best" blow job? It's easy to feel insecure with that kind of pressure.

In comparison, vulvas have gotten terrible PR. Not only do many penis owners often feel intimidated and unsure about how to please them, but many vulva owners themselves carry around genital shame that keeps them from the pleasure of receiving. I constantly hear vulva owners use words like "gross," "disgusting," and "dirty" to describe their own genitals. Of course, with those words in their heads they don't feel completely comfortable with their partner's face between their legs.

Vulva owners are also conditioned to prioritize a penis owner's pleasure over their own. A young woman recently described to me a "friends with benefits" situation that she was excited about. She told me all about how he came over, she gave him a blow job, they had sex, and then they ordered pizza.

"Sounds fun," I told her. "Did he go down on you?"

"Ew, gross, no way," she said. "I never would have let him do that. Thank God he didn't try."

"So," I asked her, "what exactly was your benefit?"

This young woman was excited to have an FWB situation because it was the first time she was friends with the guy she'd slept with, and it didn't seem like "just a hookup." But it seemed to me that it was just a hookup with pizza. There was still no pleasure to be had by her.

This is all too common. There are some exceptions, but most penis owners are happy to receive oral sex and even assume that they'll receive it, while many vulva owners are more comfortable giving oral sex than receiving. Between their blow job performance being tied to their self-worth and their deeply internalized genital shame, I understand this.

Some vulva owners also worry that they'll take "too long" to orgasm or won't be able to orgasm at all, and that their partners will get frustrated, bored, or lockjawed. I can't tell you how many times I had a guy going down on me while I snuck a look at the clock to see how many minutes had passed. I now realize that this completely took me out of the moment and brought any pleasure I was receiving to a screeching halt. It also decreased any chance I had at orgasming.

Here's the thing. Pleasure is an inside job. If you get stuck in your head, wondering why it's taking so long or worrying about whether or not you'll orgasm at all, it will become a self-fulfilling prophecy. Remember, you can't be stressed and writhing in pleasure at the same time.

Plus, so what if you don't have an orgasm, or if it takes a while? On average, vulva owners take longer to orgasm than their penis-owning partners. Oral is a great way to get closer to orgasm because it's a big part of the arousal process, but orgasms aren't the point of oral. Eroticism is, and arousal and potential orgasms are a great bonus. There's endless pleasure to be had when you relinquish your power and let a partner do something so generous for you.

Don't forget that there is also pleasure in oral sex for the giver, too. Most people enjoy and are turned on by giving their partner pleasure. It's not gross or an inconvenience. It's more often something that they truly want to do.

Because it touches on an aspect of sex that's collaborative in a very specific way—one partner giving and the other partner receiving—the key to great oral is the energy that we bring to each role, feeling comfortable and (ideally) excited in both. At the end of the day, fantastic oral sex is less about technique and way more about the emotional qualities that you bring to the experience: enthusiasm, intimacy, and vulnerability.

I dream of a world where partners equally give and receive oral sex with pleasure and confidence, and we can all relax into receiving the pleasure that's right there in front of us. So, I'm going to save my tips for giving oral until later and start with the equally important topic of receiving.

Relaxing into Oral Pleasure

There are three main areas to focus on to remove any mental blocks you may have around receiving oral. Grounded in Sex IQ, these are ways to train your mind and body to relax, receive, and experience more pleasure. They are: rewiring your brain, understanding the impact of what you put into your body, and gaining acceptance around your genitals.

Rewire Your Brain

When we talked about solo sex earlier, we looked at mindful masturbation as a ritual to enhance embodiment and get more attuned to your body's sensations of pleasure. This will also help prepare your body and brain to receive oral sex.

There's an additional tweak you can make to your mindful masturbation practice if you want to use solo sex to help you relax into pleasure during oral. As you stimulate yourself, consciously envision yourself receiving oral. Imagine that the sensations you're feeling are coming from your partner's tongue instead of your finger or vibrator.

This may be challenging at first. You might be deep into your mindful masturbation practice, picture yourself receiving oral, and suddenly feel your arousal disappear. This is frustrating, but stick with it.

The more you practice linking the image of yourself receiving oral to pleasurable sensations, the more pleasurable oral will be. You are literally tricking your brain into getting more pleasure from oral! When we are attuned to our body's cues, we can amplify our pleasure and direct it toward the kind of future experiences that we want. We get to be the designers of our own pleasure.

There is an added benefit here. When you orgasm, your brain releases dopamine, the learning and motivation hormone we discussed earlier. While we have to be careful to keep our dopamine levels balanced, it can be our ally here. Dopamine teaches our brains what feels good. By imaging yourself receiving oral while you orgasm, you are leveraging dopamine to teach your brain that receiving oral is super pleasurable.

Understand the Impact of What You Put in Your Body

Both vulva and penis owners often worry about how their genitals smell or taste and whether it will be off-putting to a partner. Here's the main thing that I want you to know about this: if you are generally in good health, your genitals will smell and taste just fine. In fact, your partner will likely find their natural smell and taste arousing. There is no need to douche or use special perfumes. These products are likely to cause infections and irritation and can disrupt the natural microbiome that keeps your vagina healthy and in balance. Bodies aren't supposed to smell like fruit or flowers. The vagina can smell or taste a bit different throughout the month, and some medications can change your natural odor. Try not to feel insecure about this or let it stand in the way of your pleasure.

With that said, there are times when things can be off. In vulva owners, one of the main culprits here is bacterial vaginosis, an infection that can cause an unpleasant odor. This is common and no big deal, and it goes away after a couple of days of antibiotics.

The problem is, many vulva owners don't realize they have bacterial vaginosis or another infection at first because their noses aren't located close to their genitals. This is one of many reasons that healthy, open communication between sex partners is so important. Many people fear that they would die of shame if their partner said their vagina didn't smell as lovely as usual. If this happens, please know that it's normal and not your fault and not any indication of how badly your partner wants you.

If you are the one who has to break this news to your partner, please remember all of the tips from the chapter on communication and include plenty of affirmation. Try something like "Babe, you always taste so good, and I love going down on you. Lately, I've noticed that something is different. It doesn't stop me from wanting you, and please try not to take it personally, but I just wanted you to know in case you want to get it checked out."

Aside from this type of infection, the main factor that can change the smell and taste of your semen or vaginal secretions is your lifestyle—specifically, what you eat and drink. The nice thing is that this is within your control, so if you have concerns about this, it's a somewhat easy fix.

I once spoke to a woman who was down for oral sex in general and had always enjoyed giving her partners blow jobs. But she found the taste of her most recent partner's semen incredibly off-putting. This wasn't a hygiene issue. He showered regularly, sometimes right before sex, and the problem persisted. She had no idea what was causing it or how to address it with him.

After asking a few other questions, I asked about her partner's lifestyle, and she told me that he ate fast food almost every day, smoked two packs of cigarettes daily, and drank a significant amount of alcohol. Well, there we had it—the answer she had been looking for. The taste of his semen was coming from the pollutants he was putting into his body.

What you consume on a daily basis can affect the scent profile of your semen or vaginal lubrication. I'm not talking about one meal or drink or even going wild on vacation. This is more about your long-term lifestyle.

Generally speaking, the substances that we know are bad for us also have the greatest impact here—cigarettes, alcohol, caffeine, and the chemicals and preservatives found in processed food. This doesn't mean that you can't have your daily coffee or a glass or two of wine or even an occasional Big Mac and still taste great. The damage is done when you consume these things in excess. In excess, meat, dairy products, and high sulfur foods like cauliflower and cabbage can also alter the taste and smell of your semen or vaginal secretions.

Of course, it's also best for your general health and well-being to avoid pretty much anything in excess. And you already know how much your overall health affects your sexual health. It's great to know that as you grow in this pillar of Sex IQ, you will also be able to feel more confident receiving oral sex, too.

Accept Your Genitals

When it comes to insecurities, our genitals usually take the cake, and that goes for vulva and penis owners alike. But feeling insecure about your genitals makes it virtually impossible for you to fully enjoy oral. It's time to kick genital shame to the curb once and for all. For many of us, this shame is deeply embedded, and healing may not be an overnight process. But with ongoing effort, it is within your reach.

So many vulva owners are either afraid to look at their vulvas because they believe that vulvas are "gross," or they are convinced that their own perfectly normal parts are ugly or misshaped. Of course, this makes them want to avoid having their partner's face up close and personal with their genitals.

We rarely look at vulvas, and if we do see them, it's in photos that were retouched or in anatomical diagrams or models that appear perfectly symmetrical with no visible inner labia. Maybe we've seen some vulvas that look one particular way in the porn we've watched and compared them to ours. However, every vulva is different. They don't come from a designer template, and we don't often see the incredible variance of vulva shapes and sizes. This makes it easy to assume there is a "right" way for our vulvas to look.

It's common to blame vulva insecurity on porn, but in reality, this insecurity stems from the fact that we've mostly received inaccurate or fear-based education about our bodies and genitals since childhood—if we received any education about them at all.

In a fascinating study, women were shown images of surgically modified vulvas and nonmodified ones. One group saw the modified vulvas before the nonmodified ones. This group rated the modified vulvas as "more normal" than the nonmodified ones. The second group who saw nonmodified vulvas first rated the modified ones as "less normal." This is profound because it shows that when we see images of surgically altered vulvas, it changes how we feel about our own bodies.

Unsurprisingly, most penis owners are also insecure about their genitals. They worry that they're too small or too curved or even too large. In reality, there is no such thing as a perfect penis, and even if there were, that perfect penis wouldn't automatically make its owner a great partner or lover.

One way for both vulva and penis owners to begin accepting their genitals is to take a look at them. Most penis owners don't need to be told to do this, but if you haven't taken a good look at your penis from every angle, grab a mirror. Don't forget to look at your testicles, too. Get to know your genitals in a new way, with no intention of having an orgasm (although if this exercise turns you on, that's okay, too).

Most vulva owners I know couldn't pick theirs out of a lineup. I highly recommend grabbing a hand mirror and exploring. Our vulvas are so complex and multifaceted. Allow yourself to be amazed by everything you've got going on down there.

It's also helpful to take a gander at more gentials to see how diverse and beautiful our bodies truly are. I love the website All Vulvas Are Beautiful, which was created by Dutch illustrator Hilde Atalanta and features beautifully illustrated artwork featuring vulvas paired with personal stories.

Similarly, artist Alexandra Rubinstein (who has a brilliant Instagram account), uses oil paints to create pieces depicting penises of all sizes and shapes. While they appear in surreal settings in her art, Rubinstein paints them from a place of loving curiosity, which is exactly how I want you to start looking at your own penis.

Ultimately, this exercise isn't about convincing yourself that your genitals are "perfect" or "the best." You're not in some sort of genital beauty contest. Instead, I want you to reach that state of neutral acceptance, knowing that your genitals are fine and normal and deserving of all the pleasure in the world.

Confidently Giving Oral Pleasure

While there are some Jacks out there who believe that giving oral isn't their thing, there are many others who adore giving their partners oral. Why? First of all, it feels good to give, especially to give to someone you love. Giving your partner oral is a way of making them feel nurtured, loved, and accepted.

It's also an act that puts you completely in control, and for many people this power dynamic is a huge turn-on. It's empowering to know that you can give your partner orgasms without them doing anything. This can help expand your erotic identity.

Ultimately, giving oral isn't a performance, a job, or a duty. It's a gift—an intimate way of connecting to another person and adding more pleasure to both of your lives.

The most important tip that I can give you to deliver mind-blowing oral sex to any type of genitals is that technique always comes secondary to enthusiasm. The energy you bring to oral is far more important than anything you do with your lips, tongue, or mouth. Think about it—how hot would it be if the person giving you oral seemed half-hearted about it? Not very. Part of the intense eroticism of oral sex is knowing that your partner wants you so badly that they crave having your genitals in their mouth. Much hotter, right?

Also keep in mind that despite any tips I give you, when you're giving oral, it is one of the most important times to focus on your partner's cues. No two people receiving oral will ever be exactly the same. What feels great to one person might be downright painful to another. Don't just hunker down thinking, "This is how Emily told me to do it!"

Try out these tips, but pay attention to what feels good to your partner. Which types of tongue movements make them moan? What are you doing when they seem to tune out or lose interest? Don't be afraid to check in with them throughout. It can be very sexy for someone to ask, "Do you like that?... How about that?"

Oral sex is a dance. Even though one partner is doing most of the work, you are still collaborating to create eroticism together. So, while I hope that these techniques help build your confidence, remember that enthusiasm and connection are the real keys.

With that said, let's get to it. Here are my best tips for how to orally please a vulva or a penis.

Performing Oral Sex on a Vulva

When going down on a vulva, the first and most important thing that you should do is put your partner at ease. They might be feeling nervous about whether or not they'll orgasm and how long it will take, how they taste and smell, and if this is something you even really want to do. Remember, the more relaxed your partner is, the more likely they are to orgasm. Before you dive in, make it clear how excited you are. "I can't wait to taste you" is sexy. So is "You just relax. I've got all night, and I'm not going anywhere."

Once you've started, it can also be really hot to pause for a moment and say something along the lines of "You taste so good." Moaning a little as you go down on them is also a great way of letting your partner know that you're enjoying it as much as they are. This will help your partner relax and enjoy what you're doing that much more.

So, what exactly should you be doing?

Step 1: The Tease

A big part of giving oral sex to a vulva is leading up to the sweet spot—the clitoris. Don't pounce on it right away. The clitoris is an incredibly sensitive piece of sexual real estate. It can be painful if you stimulate it too soon or too hard.

Build excitement first by teasing and pleasing other areas, possibly working your way downward. Maybe kiss or lightly bite your partner's neck, then lick or pinch the nipples, making eye contact as you slowly move your lips lower. Travel down their stomach until you reach the inner thighs. This is a sensitive area that's perfect for kisses or nibbles while your hands explore grabbing their thighs or touching their chest.

Once you are between their legs, continue to resist the urge to go right for the clitoris. In fact, keep their underwear on as you use your fingers to tease them above the fabric. This is a great way of building anticipation. It's also really hot to lick a little bit over the fabric, which gives a nice visual of what's to come, plus the fabric can feel really good against all those nerve endings.

Once the underwear is off, use your mouth to continue teasing around the area—the inner thighs and mons pubis. You can also insert a finger into the vagina, moving it slowly in and out.

Not everyone likes this, so ask for permission first and then try it out and watch for telltale sounds of arousal—changes in breathing, moaning, and/or moving their hips to meet you.

Step 2: Getting Closer

Now it's time to pay attention to the vulva, but not the clitoris yet. Lick the outer labia and the vaginal opening. Draw circles with your tongue around the clitoris itself.

This can be a good time to apply lube. Many people assume that lube is just for penetrative sex, but it's a must for any kind of sex. The clitoris itself doesn't self-lubricate, and the slippery sensations from lube make everything feel so much more pleasurable. I highly recommend experimenting with flavored lubes, which make oral sex more fun for the giver and receiver.

Step 3: Go for It

Finally, now is the moment they've been waiting for. Use your tongue to apply gentle pressure to the clitoris itself. Just graze it lightly to build sensation. Don't forget about your hands here. It's sexy to grip their thighs or hands while your mouth does its thing. Holding hands during oral can feel incredibly intimate and even romantic.

Allow your licks to become more forceful, paying close attention to how your partner responds. Do they react more strongly when you lick up and down or side to side? With more or less pressure? Don't be afraid to ask. Some partners also love to have their clitoris sucked, while some prefer a softer touch. Give it a shot, and see how they like it.

As you go, experiment with tongue and mouth variety: a pointed, targeted tongue, a softer, flatter tongue, a tongue moving in circles, a tongue moving up and down, and so on.

You can also try inserting a finger or two and see how they like it. This is an ideal opportunity to find their G-area, about two inches inside their vagina and press or stroke it for major stimulation. It's easier to find the G-area once you're already aroused because it becomes engorged with blood and swells.

Now it's time to be more assertive. Use your fingers to spread the labia, exposing their clitoris even more. When you put your mouth back on it, they'll feel everything more intensely.

If at some point, your mouth or jaw gets tired, take a break and go back to using your fingers to stimulate, if your partner likes it. This could also be a good time to introduce a toy, either internally or against the clitoris. If, and only if, your partner is into it, you can also try penetrating their anus with a lubed-up finger, and then add the oral stimulation back in.

Feel free to mix it up, but any point, if your partner says, "Don't stop," then by all means, keep doing exactly what you're doing. Those repetitive movements are critical when an orgasm is building.

Step 4: The Finale

If they have an orgasm, great! You can follow with penetrative sex or have your partner give you oral sex or just call it a night. All great options. However, you could try giving your partner another orgasm.

After a clitoral orgasm from oral, the internal vaginal walls will be engorged and more sensitive. If they want more, give them a break to recover with kisses on the thighs, eye contact, and more of those reassuring words. When they're ready, insert a finger or a toy to find the G-spot. If they approach orgasm again, they can bear down with their pelvic floor muscles to encourage squirting.

But remember—it's also completely okay if your partner doesn't have an orgasm at all. Orgasms aren't the goal of oral sex or of any kind of sex, really. The goal is to experience intimacy, connection, and pleasure.

Performing Oral Sex on a Penis

Here's a fun fact—in seventeenth century Europe, to "blow" meant to bring someone to orgasm. However, just like giving oral sex to a vulva, blow jobs aren't strictly about orgasms, either. Instead, this is an incredibly intimate and creative act that recipients pretty much universally love. They get to completely relax and let go of the reigns of the sexual experience, and the sensations you can give them with your mouth are ones they can't get anywhere else. If that isn't powerful, I don't know what is.

Just like vulva owners, all penis owners are different and enjoy different things. Experiment, pay close attention to their cues, and ask about what they like. As you get more attuned to their body language and vocal responses, you can get a feel for what they love.

Penis owners also benefit from plenty of affirmations and enthusiasm. Many of them internalize the phrase "blow job" and assume their partners don't enjoy giving them oral sex. It feels so much better when it's clear that the giver is enjoying it, too. "I love your dick," or "I can't wait to get you in my mouth," are good places to start. So is a little moaning during the act, which shows enthusiasm and has the benefit of creating new sensations. No matter how you choose to do it, your main goal here is to make that penis feel like it's the only thing you care about for the next several minutes.

Step 1: The Build-Up

As for the act itself, in the beginning it's not that different from giving oral sex to a vulva owner. Go slow, work your way down, and kiss your partner's chest, stomach, and inner thighs. Don't just check these off your list. Take your time to explore these areas and arouse your partner.

While you're still exploring other parts of their body with your mouth, wrap your fingers around the shaft of the penis. This is a good time to add moisture from either saliva or lube. Once again, I'll make my pitch for flavored lube, which can really heighten this experience for both of you. After it's well moistened, move your hand up and down to wake up the nerve endings along the shaft.

Step 2: The Main Act

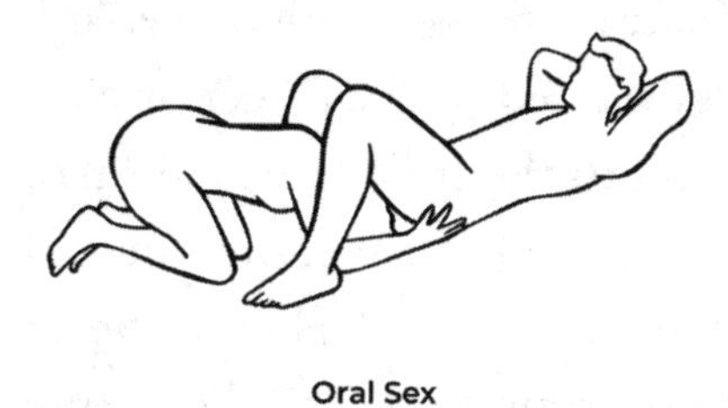

Oral Sex

Then it's time to move on to the blow job itself. Start by licking the penis with a slow, steady pace. Use your hand to continue stimulating the shaft. Next, create suction. Pull your lips in over your teeth so that you don't accidentally scrape the penis. Then envelope it with your mouth and suck—gently at first and then a little harder.

Now's a good time to tune in. How are they reacting? Is their breath changing? Are they moaning? Use these reactions for clues about what's working. You can also ask if what you're doing feels good. If you've tried mutual masturbation, which I hope you have, try to replicate the type of movements your partner used to please themselves. Those will likely feel amazing here, too.

As you continue, don't be afraid to keep using your hands. You can suck on the tip of the penis while using your hand to stroke the shaft to stimulate the entire penis. Imagine that your hand is an extension of your mouth. And you can always go back to your hands to give yourself a break if your mouth or jaw gets tired.

Step 3: Mix It Up

If you want to add some variety, try stimulating your partner's testicles. Some penis owners love this, while others find it too sensitive. To try it out, hold their testicles in one hand while you stimulate their penis with your mouth, gently massaging the testicles in your hand. You can also take a break from the penis itself or switch to your hand and stimulate the testicles with your mouth. Try using your tongue to make swirls around each one.

Another variation is to use a hand to apply light pressure to the perineum while stimulating your partner's penis with your mouth (and maybe a hand). This area is packed with nerves and feels good when gently stroked or pressed with a finger or two.

Also remember to pay attention to the frenulum, the small tag of skin on the underside of the penis, between the foreskin and the shaft. As a nerve-dense region, it can feel amazing to some penis owners to have this area stimulated. Try alternating between slow and fast licks.

It can also be fun to add a toy to the mix during a blow job. Place a vibrator against the shaft and then lick or suck the tip of the penis. Holding a vibrator against the perineum feels great to many penis owners, too. You can even hold a vibrator against your cheek or under your chin, and your partner will feel it on the penis!

As you progress, go from lighter to harder suction and faster stroking to get your partner closer to orgasm.

Step 4: The Finale

When they are getting close, apply more pressure, not less, and continue stimulation all the way through orgasm and ejaculation. If you don't want them to come in your mouth, ask your partner to tell you when they're going to come, and then finish them off with your hand.

Speaking of which, use those communication skills to plan ahead on where you want your partner to ejaculate, whether it's in your mouth, somewhere on your body, or in your hand. If you really have no preference, it can be hot to ask your partner, "Where do you want to come?"

Some penis owners like to receive oral as a form of foreplay. For others, it's all about the intimacy and acceptance that comes with the act. And blow jobs are a great way of enhancing connection and arousal. Let go of the pressure and focus on the pleasure.

To Deep Throat or Not To Deep Throat

Always remember that the sex you see in porn is almost always unrealistic—and that includes the oral sex. In porn, we often see partners "deep throating" their partner's penis, meaning they take the entire penis into their mouth, until it's in their throat. Some porn stars are famous for this, but for many people it can trigger the gag reflex and be very uncomfortable.

Sure, some penis owners love getting deep throated, and some givers like to do it. But it can be difficult, especially if the penis in question is on the bigger side. Watching porn might give you the impression that this is an essential part of giving a good blow job, but that's not true, and it's not necessary for you to do it unless you want to. (Of course, that goes for every other sex act, too.)

If, and only if, you want to try deep throating and/or your gag reflex is a bit too active while giving blow jobs in general, you can work to relax it. Every day, after you brush your teeth, place the toothbrush on your tongue and hold it down for five seconds. Move it a bit further back on your tongue each day, and hold it down for a little longer. This helps get your mouth and throat muscles used to having something in there without you choking on it. Given time, it will adjust.

Until then, or if you have no interest in deep throating, or if your partner doesn't want it, rest assured that it's more than possible to give a fantastic blow job without adding this little trick.

Oral Sex Positions

The go-to standard oral sex position has the receiver lying on their back and the giver lying or kneeling between their legs.

That's all fine and great, but there are plenty of other positions that you can try, too. Each provide slightly different access and sensations, so it's always good to experiment and see which ones you and your partner like best.

As the giver, it's especially important to make yourself comfortable. If giving your partner oral sex feels like a job, make it less of a job! At any point, if one position becomes difficult to hold, switch it up and try something else. This is also a great way of continuing to create new sensations throughout your oral sex session. Here are some good ones to try:

The Pillow Position

To give a vulva owner oral sex, place a pillow or two underneath your partner's hips. There are also sex pillows you can buy that are made specifically to tilt their hips upward, giving your better access to the vulva and the anus.

Doggy Style

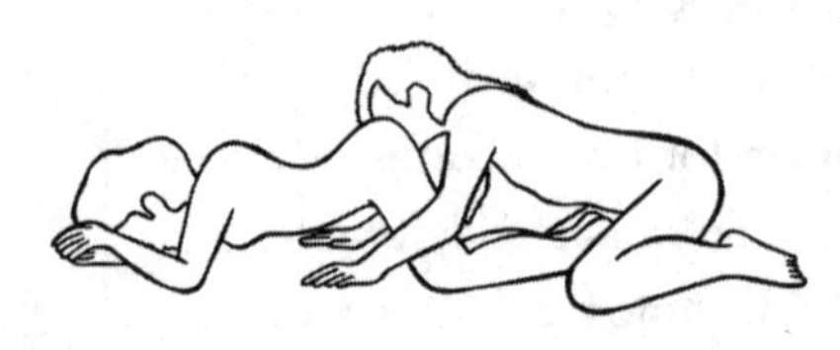

Doggy Style Oral

Try going down on your vulva owning partner from behind. This is especially handy (no pun intended) if your partner is into a little anal play.

Face Sitting

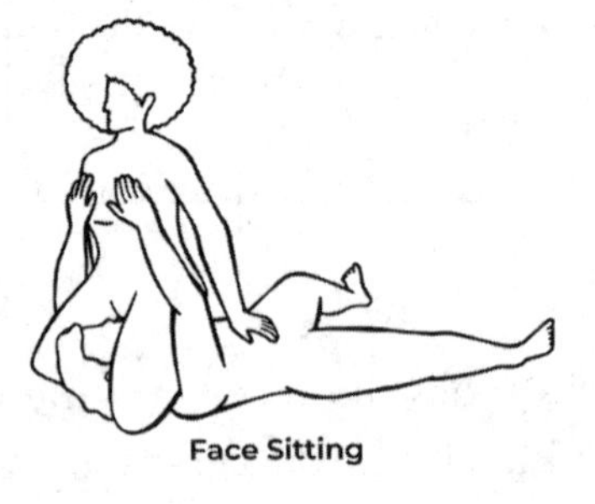

Face Sitting

This position might be better called Face Kneeling than Face Sitting, because kneeling gives you more leverage. Plus, some people feel that the term Face Sitting feels too aggressive.

That said, this position can work for vulva and penis owners alike. Lie on your back and have your partner straddle your chest and scoot forward until their genitals meet your mouth. This is a fun position because it gives you great access to the rest of their body for touching and grabbing. It also gives your partner a little more control, which can be a hot way to mix things up.

Chair Sitting

In this position, your partner sits in a chair or on a couch while you kneel between their legs. A chair gives you more leverage and stability, and it's nice to get out of the bedroom. Make sure to put a pillow under your knees for added comfort. Try this one in a variety of locations around the house, especially in front of a mirror. The added visual can be really stimulating.

If you're going down on a vulva in this position, spread the labia for more clitoral exposure. If you're going down on a penis, ask about angles. Some penis owners like having the penis stretched further away from their body, some decidedly do not.

69

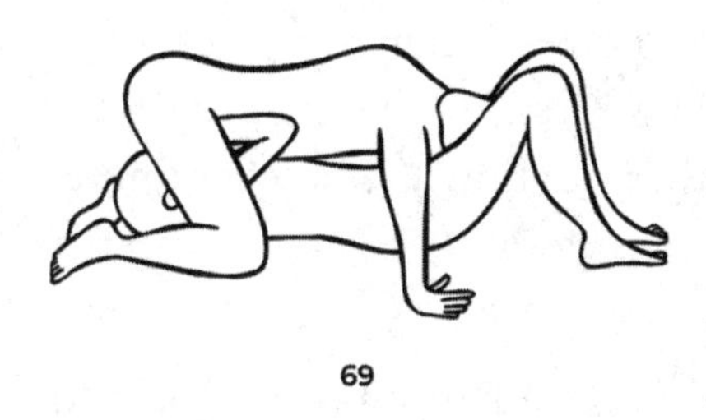

69

The great multitasker of oral sex, 69 is a real opportunity to collaborate. This position works best when you and your partner lie side by side so that you both have good mobility and visibility. A good tip here is to choose a pacesetter ahead of time. When one partner starts to lick faster or harder, the other usually takes it as a signal that they want them to speed up, too. But this can be confusing. So, choose one of you to be the pacesetter beforehand. The other partner will match their intensity and speed.

Also feel free to take turns in this position. It doesn't have to be strictly simultaneous. Go down on your partner for a few minutes, and then switch. This is a great way to practice edging, as you repeat the cycle of tease, buildup, and eventual release.

You can also add toys into the mix. The idea of 69 is to mutually give and receive pleasure, but there's no rule that says it can only be oral pleasure. As long as everyone is having fun, it's fine to cycle in hands, fingers, and toys.

Side note: some people don't like this position at all. Personally, I always wanted to either focus on giving or receiving but not both at the same time. Once I realized that it didn't have to only be my mouth doing the giving, I was able to really collaborate in a most excellent 69 session.

Standing

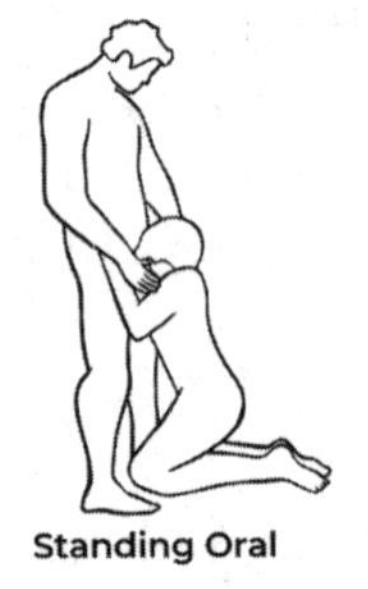
Standing Oral

When the receiving partner stands and the giver kneels between their legs, it creates a dramatic power dynamic that some people find really hot. Note that this tends to work better when going down on a penis owner, as you don't get a lot of access to a vulva in this position. But it's always worth a try, and you can switch to another position after a few minutes.

The Kivin Method

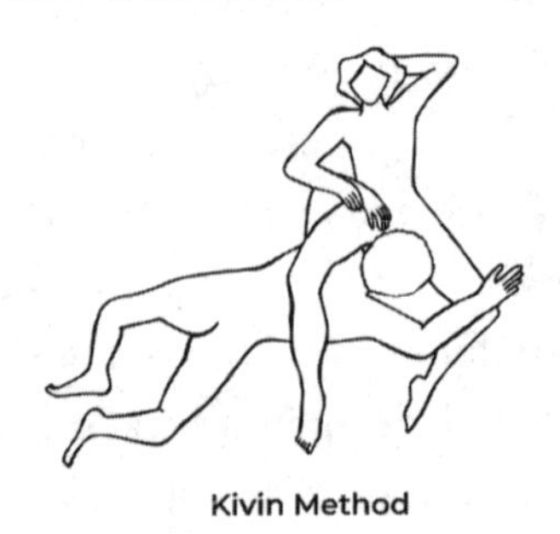
Kivin Method

I saved possibly the best for last—at least when it comes to going down on a vulva. After I talked about this on my show, I got an overwhelming response. No one really knows where this technique came from or how it got its name, but I do know many vulva owners who came thanks to it. The Kivin method is extremely powerful and definitely lives up to the hype.

Also called sideways oral, this method has the receiving partner lying on their back and the giver lying on their stomach, perpendicular to their partner's body. In other words, you are approaching the vulva from the side. This way, you're accessing and stimulating a wider area of the clitoris, including all of those tucked-in nerve endings that are harder to reach in other positions. This can help vulva owners orgasm far more powerfully and much more quickly.

To give you the best access, your partner can drape a leg over your shoulder. Then you lick from side to side instead of up and down. Use your whole tongue instead of just the tip, varying the pressure and speed to see what your partner likes.

You can also switch up positioning yourself on the left or right side. This can make a huge difference in the level of sensitivity and response. Sometimes, this positioning reveals two small bumps on either side of the clitoral hood, known as "K points." If you can feel them, use your tongue to gently sweep across these sensitive areas. But don't stress if you can't find them—not all bodies have detectable K points.

At the end of the day, no matter what position or technique you use, the best oral sex is going to have three essential ingredients: communication, collaboration, and plenty of lube. If you have those, you can rest assured that you're going to be able to give your partner amazing amounts of pleasure.

Ask for More

Like all sex acts, oral requires a lot of communication—specifically when it comes to soliciting and giving feedback and asking for more of it.

We often get frustrated because our partner doesn't know what they are doing during oral or it just doesn't feel good, but remember that you are the best advocate for your own pleasure. Oral sex should be collaborative and interactive—especially when you're with a new partner.

Speak up and figure it out together. Ask your partner what they want and what they like, and tell them what you want and what you like. Giving and receiving feedback is how we can all become oral sex experts. Let's all stop wasting precious pleasure time with the silence and politeness and go into oral knowing that it's going to take some tweaking, fine-tuning, advanced collaboration (and lube) to make this most coveted sex act the hottest it can be.

Now let's talk about getting some of that good oral to begin with. A lot (and I mean a *lot*) of people come to me for advice on how to ask their partners for more oral sex. All of the communication tips from Chapter 4 apply, but here I'll give you a few examples for how to ask based on your partner's specific issue with oral. Of course, this requires you to use those communication skills to talk about it beforehand and find out what the issue is.

The most important thing here is to approach the conversation from a place of curiosity and without judgment. Partners who are less than excited to give oral probably have their own reasons. Maybe they've had a bad experience with it or have been told that it's gross or dirty or wrong.

Many vulva owners have been conditioned to think that only "sluts" and "whores" give blow jobs, or that giving one makes them subservient and goes against their feminist values. Likewise, many penis owners have heard that going down on a vulva will make them "less of a man." These are all ridiculous, but they are all myths that have circulated in our culture and are often deeply ingrained.

Regardless of the reason, part of being in an intimate relationship is having difficult conversations to better understand where our partners are coming from. Here are a few sample scripts you can use to tackle common mental blocks around oral. Communication is personal, and these may feel awkward or unnatural to you, so please feel free to make them your own.

If your partner has had a bad past experience with oral sex: "The idea of you going down on me is such a turn-on, and I want to give it to you, too. I know it hasn't been so hot for you in the past. Can we talk about what turned you off? I'd love to better understand so we can work together to turn it into something we both love."

If your partner associates it with something dirty, gross, or unhygienic: "I totally hear you. Growing up, I was also told that oral sex was disgusting, but I think that was more about people's fears and ignorance around sex in general. I'd love to create a new association with it. Would you be open to learning more about it with me? We could watch some ethical porn together and see if it turns us on. I'd love to evolve oral into a sexy idea for both of us. It could even be hot to shower together beforehand."

If your partner doesn't enjoy it: "I get your hesitation. I wouldn't want to do something in bed that I didn't like, either. But maybe if we talked about what you don't like about it, we could make some adjustments. We could add a toy or some flavored lube to the mix, or find a position that's more comfortable. Are you up for experimenting with me?"

More than anything else, oral sex is a conduit for our eroticism. As a unique and incredibly intimate sexual experience, oral sex allows us to collaborate with our partners and experiment with power and polarity through defined roles of giving and receiving. This leads us perfectly to the next chapter, where we'll continue to play with all of these aspects of sex in a variety of positions.

7

Reassume the Positions:

Intentional, Collaborative, Penetrative Sex

Not only did I used to fake all of my orgasms, but for the first several years of my sex life, sex for me was almost completely performative. I assumed that sex was supposed to feel good automatically, and when it didn't, I thought there was something wrong with me. I didn't want anyone to find out, so instead of getting curious and exploring my own body, collaborating with my partners, or being honest about what I did and didn't enjoy, I did what many people in the same situation do—I put on a show.

I was so determined to convince my partners that I was loving sex that eventually I got really good at pretending. I emulated what I'd seen in porn, tossing my hair around and moaning and screaming. The irony of this is that the very thing I was trying to recreate wasn't real, either. People in porn are acting, too. And there I was, performing sex for an audience of one instead of fully experiencing or deriving pleasure from it. Of course, this only kept me stuck in my own lie, unable to explore and discover what actually felt good to me.

If you've been "performing" sex rather than having fully embodied and pleasurable sex, I hope that by now you're starting to work your way out of this trap. Maybe you've begun a mindful masturbation practice and started to tune in to what brings you pleasure. Maybe you're working to become more embodied. Maybe you've opened a conversation with your partner about sex. Or maybe you've started the work of identifying and releasing some of your mental hang-ups around sex in general or certain sex acts.

These are all amazing and transformative steps. Even if you haven't taken any action at all yet, trust that by absorbing all of the information you've read so far, you are also well on your way to deriving pleasure that is your birthright.

The next step is to begin reimagining what penetrative sex can and should be.

Penetrating Self-Awareness

Of course, penetrative sex can involve any types of partners with any types of genitals. Throughout this chapter, I'll refer to a penetrating partner and a receiving partner, but these can be partners of any gender, with or without a penis or the assistance of a strap-on or dildo. Here I'm referring to vaginal sex specifically, but you don't have to commit to one role or the other throughout your entire sexual career. Many partners enjoy switching roles and trying out being the penetrator or receiver from time to time.

Penetrating the Routine

When it comes to penetrative sex we all know the basic positions. After all, there are only so many ways to insert Tab A into Slot B, right? You might have your favorite go-to position or enjoy working your way through a series of positions during each sexual experience.

Some people know which position will get them or their partner off quickly and stick to it when they don't have a lot of time or energy. Many know which one works when they want to feel more connected to their partner and revert to that when they're needing closeness. And some people know which position helps them last the longest and go for that one when they want a marathon session.

That's all great. Good information to have! The potential problem here, though, is muscle memory. When we repeat any type of physical task, our neurons learn exactly how to do it without our brains having to start from scratch and send instructions to our muscles every time. This is great for efficiency, but not ideal for enhancing pleasure.

Due to this muscle memory, after a while, our bodies start to do things the same ways as always, and that habituated response keeps us less attuned. Even when we don't intend for it to happen, our bodies start just going through the motions. When it comes to sex in general, forced sameness can feel comforting and safe, but it can also limit our pleasure. It's novelty that wakes up our neurons and makes our bodies more sensitive and receptive, in part because they're not relying on the muscle memory that makes things feel routine. We're also forced to be present when we're doing something new.

The good news is that with a few small tweaks, what was once stale and routine can feel brand-new and exciting again. In the end, penetrative sex is not as simple as "insert here." In fact, there is an endless variety of new sensations just waiting to be discovered, even in familiar positions.

It's also possible that you think you've explored many different sex positions but haven't fully experienced the multiple nuances and potential depths of pleasure in each. After all, we only know our own experiences. No one teaches us how to angle our hips in one position to maximize G-area access or to put a pillow under our knees to make a formerly uncomfortable and dreaded position suddenly much more comfortable and pleasurable.

I want to help you make these positions feel more intentional and less automatic with both big and small changes. At the same time, I'll provide opportunities to enhance your collaboration, self-knowledge, and pleasure in each position.

Don't be afraid to make each position your own. Find angles that work for you and adjust your rhythm. It's also common to move really fast as a default, so remember to slow down. Focus on your breath and stay attuned to the sensations you're feeling. This will help you figure out how to adjust positions so they feel as good as possible for you.

Penetrating Our Preferences

Of course, some positions will feel better to each of us physically, largely due to how our individual bodies are built. But there is much more to different sex positions than physical sensations. Exploring different positions to see which ones feel best to us can help us understand who we are and what we need as sexual beings. This is a powerful way of growing our self-knowledge IQ pillar.

Some positions offer us the intimacy of eye contact. Others give us a chance to play around with power dynamics. And some we enjoy because we know exactly what we need to do to have an orgasm. Instead of doing the same old things out of habit or even making my suggested tweaks and getting on with it, it is well worth taking some time to consider what aspect of some positions give you a sexual charge and, most important, *why*.

For example, if you have hesitations about having sex from behind, consider what specifically about that position gives you pause. Some recipients miss the intimacy of eye contact in this position. Some like having their bodies less on display, while others may feel objectified in this position. All of these factors can be a turn-on for some people and a turn-off for others.

We can only open our minds (and bodies) to new forms of pleasure once we understand what may be keeping us from fully experiencing them to begin with. This doesn't mean that you have to start loving every position. Exactly the opposite! It's empowering to be able to say, "I know and understand what I like and what I don't, and I'm going to grow with it and do more of what brings me pleasure."

However, penetrative sex is one sex act that's definitely not all about you. Everything that you do to make different sex positions more pleasurable will involve some level of collaboration. In fact, Sex IQ pillar #3, Collaboration, is extremely important during penetrative sex.

Penetrative sex is literally a give-and-take between a giver and a recipient, but it is nowhere near as simple as one partner being active while the other is passive. Every sex position is really about what you and your partner each bring to it. A position with rear entry can feel taboo and sometimes laden with power dynamics, or it can feel really sweet and even romantic. It all depends on the energy that you both bring to the experience and the sexual mood that you co-create together.

This means that you might love having sex in a certain position with one partner and feel deeply uncomfortable (physically and/or emotionally) in the exact same position with someone else. Again, it is important here to understand why. What is it about how your bodies, minds, and energies are working together that makes this position feel more or less pleasurable for you?

Penetrating Shame

One Pleasure Thief that keeps so many people from fully enjoying certain positions is shame—body shame in particular. It can get really complicated when shame about penetrative sex positions gets wrapped up with our upbringings, expectations, and body insecurities.

Some positions are more revealing than others, and it's common to avoid those positions completely; insist on only having sex with the lights off; or get in your head, wondering if your butt or belly is jiggling and if that is a turn-off for your partner. If this is you, accept that this is where you are right now and commit to working on your self-acceptance. I promise that the problem isn't jiggle—it's shame. And once you are aware of it, you can work through it.

One way to begin navigating your shame is to disclose it. Tell your partner, "I love having sex with you, and I want to please you. But I have some insecurities that are blocking me." If the thought of saying something like this to your partner is terrifying, think about how it feels to continue to live a life devoid of real pleasure. Intimacy comes from expressing your vulnerabilities, and with deeper intimacy comes greater pleasure. When you look at it that way, our insecurities are opportunities for more pleasure.

Plus, it's incredibly liberating to speak your truth. The very second that you say the words "I'm afraid that if we have sex from behind, you won't be attracted to me anymore because of my big ass," you will be halfway to freeing yourself from that anxiety. You'll also be a lot closer to your partner. I would be willing to bet that one of the reasons they chose you is *because* of your glorious curves, and that they're dying to take you from behind.

If you're not comfortable trying a certain position, you can try other mitigating strategies. You can wear a piece of clothing or lingerie that makes you feel more confident. If you're not loving your stomach, wear something that covers you enough so that you can focus on moving in a way that feels good to you. Or cover your partner's eyes with a blindfold. When we cut off one of our senses, it enhances the others. Your partner will feel everything more intensely, and you'll be more present if you're not worrying about their gaze.

Shame and anxiety about our bodies can lead us to avoid being physically close to our partners. This can also decrease our sexual satisfaction and our ability to be present in the moment and to pay attention to our partner and their needs. Think about it this way—if you're in your head during sex, feeling anxious or worried, then the blood is rushing to your head and away from your genitals. Do what you need to do to feel more confident and present. And hopefully your pleasure and your partner's will help you get rid of that body shame for good.

As we work our way through the following positions, we will discuss their pros and cons, and ways to evolve them to make them more pleasurable.

The Big Six

These are the are most well-known and popular sex positions for a simple reason—they work. They're more than just tried and true. They're classic. Some may be slightly physically challenging, but none of them require superhuman strength and agility. And people with all types of genitals generally find them pleasurable and satisfying.

Missionary

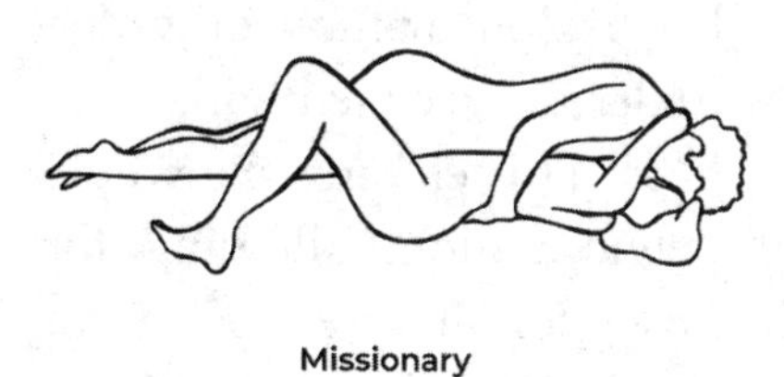

Missionary

The Basics: In the classic missionary position, the receiving partner lies on their back with the giving partner on top as they face each other. Through pop culture and its long religious legacy, missionary has often been modeled as the primary sex position.

The Pros: People who love missionary generally enjoy the full body contact and potential for eye contact and kissing during sex. Many receivers find it relaxing to lie back and let their partners take control, while givers often like being able to set the pace and intensity.

If you love missionary, it's possible that you steer toward what is safe and within your comfort zone. There's nothing wrong with that. It's up to you to consider if this is helping you have the best sex possible. If not, consider mixing it up with different positions. Our brains perk up when we try new things, so a break in routine blazes new pleasure pathways.

The Cons: There are a few downsides to missionary. The positioning itself implies gender roles that may or may not suit your sexual personality. Some people also find it easy to disassociate, or detach from the moment, in this position. When this happens, many of our Sex IQ pillars suffer. Disassociation is the opposite of presence. And pleasure, as we've discussed, is presence.

On a physical level, missionary provides minimal G-area and clitoral stimulation for vulva owners. I wish I could destroy all of those images we see of vulva owners lying on their backs and orgasming after thirty seconds of missionary. They are completely unrealistic and have led to such false expectations!

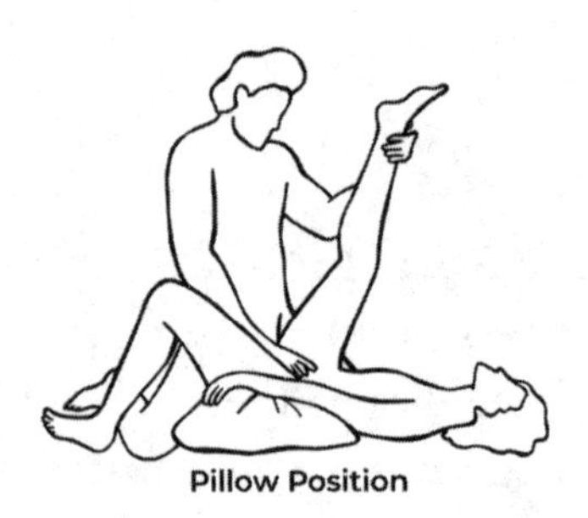

Pillow Position

The Evolution: There are tweaks that can help make missionary more exciting. You can use a vibrator or fingers to stimulate the clitoris. It also helps to put a pillow or wedge under the recipient's hips and butt. This elevates the whole pelvic region, allowing for more clitoral access, and is a great hack for almost all positions. It also makes it easier for the penis to hit the front wall of the vagina and insert deeper, giving the G-area the attention it deserves.

Another good way to mix up traditional missionary is for the recipient to lift their legs and rest them on their partner's shoulders, wrap them around their waist, bend them in toward their own chest, or put them up in the air over their head for really deep penetration. Play around and see what feels best to you and your partner.

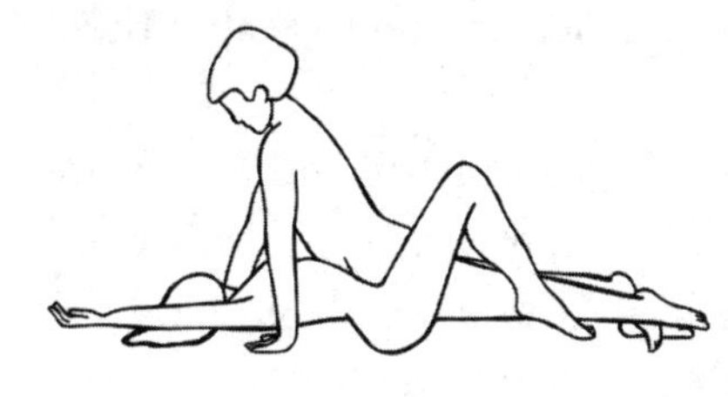

CAT: Coital Alignment Technique

The CAT: This is a version of missionary called coital alignment technique. You start CAT from missionary and match each partner's body positioning so that the penetrating partner is positioned slightly higher than usual. Have the penetrating partner scoot up a few inches over the receiver, so that the both of you can align pelvis to pelvis.

From here, create a steady rocking or grinding motion, rather than a "thrust." Take it slow, so as to stimulate the clitoris, rather than a rapid in-and-out. The focus should be on the clitoris hitting the base of the penis or mons pubis if the giver is wearing a strap-on. With this tweak, the vulva owner is going to feel a lot more sensation and potentially more orgasms because more external nerve endings are being stimulated.

Cowgirl (or Cowboy)

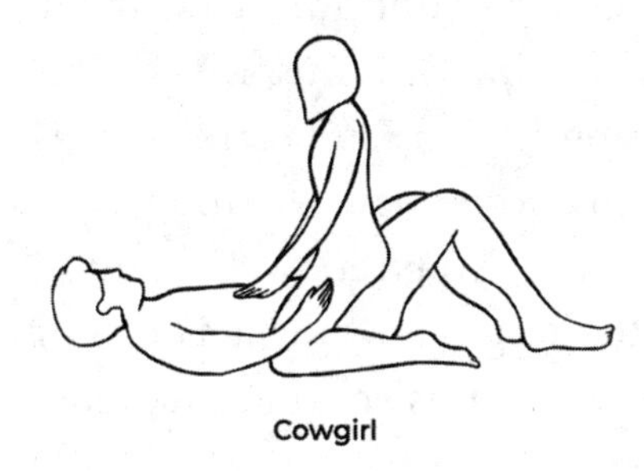

Cowgirl

The Basics: In this position, the giving partner is lying on their back, while the receiving partner straddles and "rides" them.

The Pros: This is one position where the receiving partner is in charge, controlling the pace. This can feel fresh and hot for those who are used to being more submissive, and is a nice change of pace for those who are used to being on top.

Another major aspect of cowgirl is how much the receiving partner is on display. If you're the giver, watching your partner control the pace and depth of their pleasure is hot as hell. It can be just as exciting for the partner on top to watch them watch you.

If you're a recipient that loves this position, maybe you've got a little bit of exhibitionist in you. As a giver, loving this position probably means that you're highly visual and/or enjoy letting your partner take charge.

Physically, this position makes deep insertion and G-area stimulation possible. Hooray! And if the vulva owner bears down and leans forward a little, they can grind their clitoris into their partner's pubic bone and even reach orgasm that way. They can also lean back and make space to stimulate the clitoris with hands or a toy. Vulva owners report to have more orgasms in this position because they can control the depth, speed, and angles of the penetration.

The Cons: One downside to this position is that it does require a lot of stamina from the partner who's doing the riding, and it might be tricky to find the right rhythm.

Additionally, if you're a recipient (meaning you're on top in this position) and you're still working on your self-acceptance, this position can be a challenge. If you're uncomfortable being on display, keep your bra or a cute tank or camisole on. This way, cowgirl can be a tease that builds tension before you remove everything and move on to another less revealing position. It might even be healing to try this position. Of course, self-acceptance is an inside job, but seeing how turned on your partner is by watching you might make this position a lot more comfortable and pleasurable.

The Evolution: As the recipient, once you climb on board, don't just start bobbing up and down. Take a moment to adjust your positioning. Take a few moments, actually. Many of us default toward fast sex, but we learn to be more present and embodied during slower sex. Make sure there isn't too much pressure on your knees, and see if it feels better to scooch forward or backward a bit. Sex is not a choreographed ballet with perfect precision. Get comfortable first, and then get the party started.

Once you get going, if you find yourself getting tired, try switching up the movement. Bobbing up and down can wear out those glutes. Swiveling your hips and grinding on your partner gives those muscles a break and might feel better, too, because these motions better stimulate the clitoris. The giving partner can also give you a rest by taking control of the rhythm and thrusting from the bottom. Then all you have to do is hold yourself upright.

Tip—this position makes it easy to transition to one of my favorite oral sex positions, face sitting, which you read about earlier. The receiving partner simply moves up toward the penetrating partner's face and kneels down gently over their mouth. It can be fun to try edging by going back and forth between these two positions.

Reverse Cowgirl (or Cowboy)

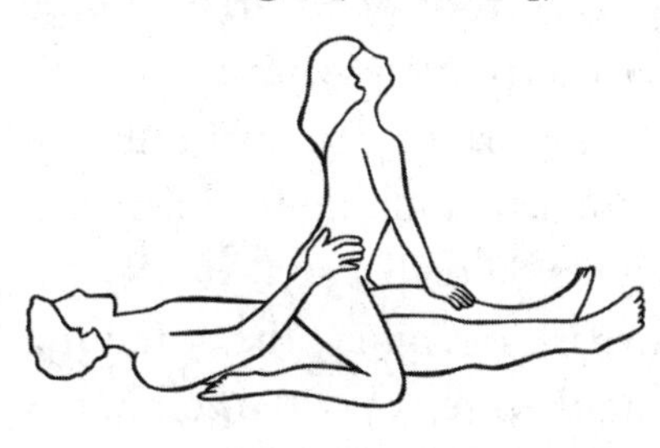

Reverse Cowgirl

The Basics: This position is just like regular cowgirl/cowboy, except that the receiving (top) partner faces backward, away from the giving partner's face.

The Pros: A major highlight here is the full moon view for the penetrating partner (and for receiving partners who like to show off their booties). This may be more comfortable for some recipients than giving a full top view. Reverse cowgirl is also a good option for pregnant receivers since there's plenty of room for a growing belly.

Like in regular cowgirl, the receiving partner sets the rhythm, which can be a turn-on for both partners. Or the giving partner can place their hands on their partner's hips and guide the movement. Reverse cowgirl also has the advantage of G-area stimulation while providing access for either partner to stimulate both the clitoris and the testicles during insertion. Many vulva owners say this is the one position in which they can feel the G-area being stimulated.

This position can also ease some anxiety during sex if face-to-face positions feel a bit too emotionally intense or if you feel self-conscious about your orgasm face. In this position, it might feel nice to close your eyes and get lost in your body's sensations. On the other hand, if you feel disconnected from your partner while facing away (and if you're flexible), you can make intermittent eye contact with a sexy glance over your shoulder.

The Cons: A lot of people are intrigued by this position, but it can be a tricky one to master. The giving partner enters the receiving partner from underneath and behind, which can put them in a precarious situation and can be uncomfortable or even dangerous. It's rare, but certain angles can strain penile tissue.

The view here is also less exciting for the receiving partner (unless they're into feet). Trying it in front of a mirror can be fun because the receiving partner can participate in the visual. We don't talk enough about how important visual stimulation is for all genders. Studies have found that looking in a mirror is often a big turn-on for vulva owners. Worth a try!

The Evolution: To reduce your risk of injury, the receiving partner can lean back a bit, bracing themselves with their hands on the bed. This ensures that the penis doesn't bend too far forward. Then you can work together to find the right rhythm. It's easiest if the receiving partner has three or four points of contact to the bed: both shins, and at least one hand. This will help with balance and stamina.

To enhance stimulation, there are a lot of options here. The giving partner can prop themselves up a bit and use a hand to reach around and stimulate the clitoris (or a penis if the receiving partner has one) with a hand or a vibrator. Of course, this position also gives plenty of access for receivers who enjoy anal play. And the receiving partner can simply reach down and play with their partner's testicles for extra stimulation.

A fun twist on this position is to practice it on the edge of the bed or a chair. In this position, the giving partner sits down with their feet touching the floor. The receiving partner sits on their lap facing away from them.

Although it doesn't offer the same view for penetrators, many people prefer this variation. It keeps you both nice and close, offering lots of skin-to-skin contact and making it easy to play with nipples and the clitoris. It also keeps the penis in a safer position, allowing penetrators to comfortably relax and enjoy.

Troubleshooting: Penis Popping

Sex is not perfect. It's not a fashion shoot, with every hair in place. It's not all that serious, either. It's messy and fun and silly, with funny sights, sounds, and smells. Instead of being embarrassed by them, embrace the awkward moments. They are bound to happen. If you can accept their inevitability, vagina farts, copious fluids, and disobedient penises will become more comic than tragic. When people ask me if they're doing sex wrong, I say, "If you're worried about doing it right, you're doing it wrong."

One common technical difficulty during penetrative sex is penis slippage, when the penis accidentally pops out of the vagina. This can happen at any time in any position, and it's no one's fault. It does not mean that the penis is too small or the vagina is too big or that either of you are doing something wrong. It's simply the result of the angle of entry and speed of movement.

If it happens to you, who cares? Make light of it,

laugh together, and switch to a different position or just add some lube and get that penis back in there. Keep in mind that a slow grind, swivel, or back-and-forth motion is less likely to cause slippage than moving up and down.

In positions like cowgirl or reverse cowgirl, it may also help to create a ninety-degree angle. You can even place a hand where your bodies meet to make sure the penis stays inside and add some manual stimulation while you're at it.

Potential penis slippage is also a good reason to slow things down. Moving slowly makes slippage much less likely to happen. When you're building momentum and getting into a rhythm, the natural impulse is to speed up for more friction. To prevent slippage, resist that urge. If you really need to move faster, switch to a less likely penis popping position, like missionary.

Rear Entry

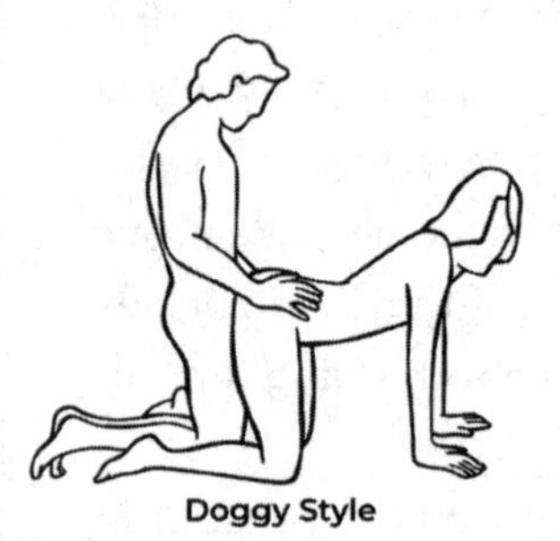

Doggy Style

The Basics: This is normally referred to as "doggy style," but I don't love that name. To me, it feels outdated and degrading, so I'm rebranding it as rear entry. Whatever you call it, this is a wildly popular position that has the receiving partner propped up on their hands and knees (or elbows and knees) while the giving partner enters their vagina from behind.

The Pros: Many people like this position because of its inherent power dynamics. The setup suggests that the giving partner is dominant while the receiving partner is more submissive. Of course, this same dynamic can be a detraction for recipients who like to be more dominant or givers who like to be more submissive. It may be worth considering your personal feelings about this position and what that might mean about your sexual energy and preferences.

This is another position that has partners facing away from each other. You might like this if eye contact during sex is intimidating or if you're a receiving partner that feels more comfortable showing off your booty than your front. For those in the penetrating position, rear entry offers a great view.

This position also makes deep insertion possible with a good angle for G-area or prostate stimulation. Of course, it's also a great position for anal play or for the giving partner to reach around and stimulate the clitoris with fingers or a toy.

The Cons: In addition to no eye contact, there isn't a lot of skin-to-skin contact in this position, either. Sometimes, this makes it feel less intimate than other positions. Consider if these factors are a turn-on or a turn-off for you and why.

This is a deep insertion position, which can be a great thing. But if the penis in question is on the bigger side, it can be painful for the recipient. If you're having this problem, try slowing way, way down and/or "shallowing," which means the penetrator doesn't insert the entire penis. Collaboration is key here. Make sure to check in with each other regularly to make sure that everything feels good.

I'm sorry to report that this is the position that is most likely to cause a penile fracture. If the penis misses the vaginal or anal opening and smashes against the partner's body at a certain speed, force and angle, the hard erectile tissue can fracture. Ouch. The result is swelling, pain, and bruising, and sometimes surgery to repair damaged tissue. Keep in mind that though it's called a "fracture," there is no bone in the penis. What's fracturing instead is engorged columns of spongey tissue, and most cases are able to heal on their own. But the only way to find out if it simply needs ice and rest or something more involved like surgery, is to go to a hospital. If left untreated, this could cause complications for the penis owner. If you even suspect a fracture, go to the hospital.

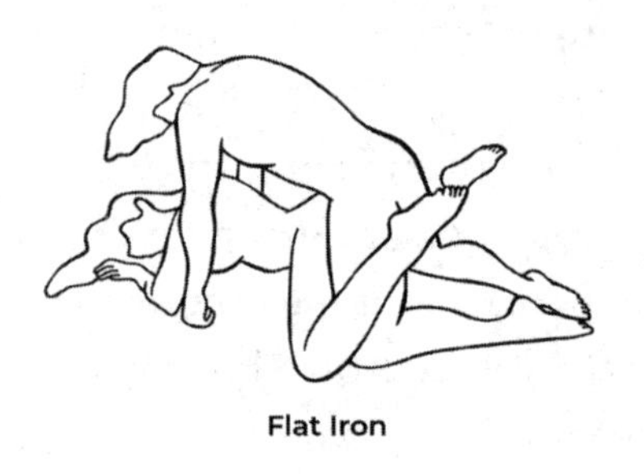
Flat Iron

The Evolution: One way to make rear entry feel more comfortable is to make the angles a little less dramatic. Have both partners stand while the receiving partner leans forward against a stable surface (my preferred shower sex position). Think hands braced against a countertop or even hands braced on the wall in front of you. This gentler bend at the hips can reduce the likelihood of the giving partner going in *too* deeply.

The receiving partner can also take control by backing up against their partner while they hold their hips in place. You can also modify the intensity by leaning all the way forward with a pillow underneath you as your partner slips in between your legs. This helps change up the position and can give the giving partner a break from aggressive thrusting.

Another nice tweak on rear entry is called flat iron. Here, the receiving partner lies flat on their belly while the giver enters them from behind. A downside here is the lack of access to the clitoris and higher potential for penis popping. This may be better for receivers who prefer anal play or simply deep insertion.

Spooning

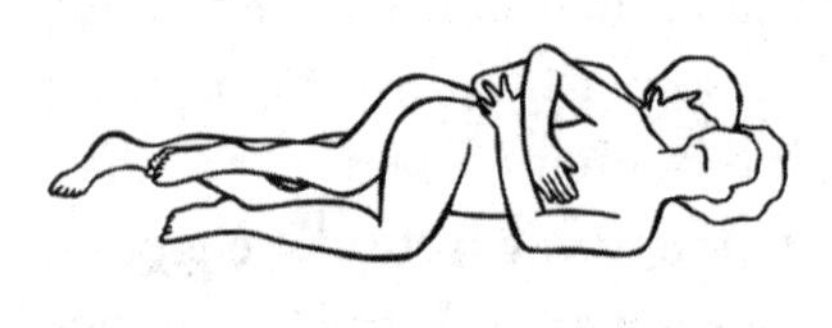
Spooning

The Basics: In this position, both partners are lying down on their sides in the classic cuddle position, and the penetrating partner enters from behind.

The Pros: This can be a very comforting position. Both people get to lie down and have lots of skin-to-skin contact, so it feels intimate even though you're not facing each other. Eye contact is possible here, though, if the receiving partner turns their head and the penetrator props themselves up on one elbow to look down at them. And don't forget the power of a mirror.

If you're on your feet all day or you're just tired and don't have the energy for a more demanding position, it's nice to have an option that is sexy and relaxing at the same time. I mean, who else here isn't ready for reverse cowgirl before coffee in the morning?

Spooning is a popular choice for pregnant bodies because it allows room for the tummy. Another nice thing about this position is that it can sneak up on you. If you're cuddling in bed or on the couch underneath a blanket, it can suddenly turn into something much hotter.

If you are a big fan of spooning, it can mean that you are looking for a particularly comforting sexual experience. Perhaps your current partner makes you feel nurtured—or maybe that's exactly what's lacking in your relationship and you're in the need of some TLC. It's also possible that spooning just hits the right buttons for you physically.

The Cons: As warm and fuzzy as this position is, it can also be an awkward one. In most other sex positions, there's a surface to bear down on. Not here. Without that, it can be a bit difficult to thrust and develop a good rhythm together. Leg positioning can also be tricky and uncomfortable, and spooning doesn't allow for particularly deep insertion.

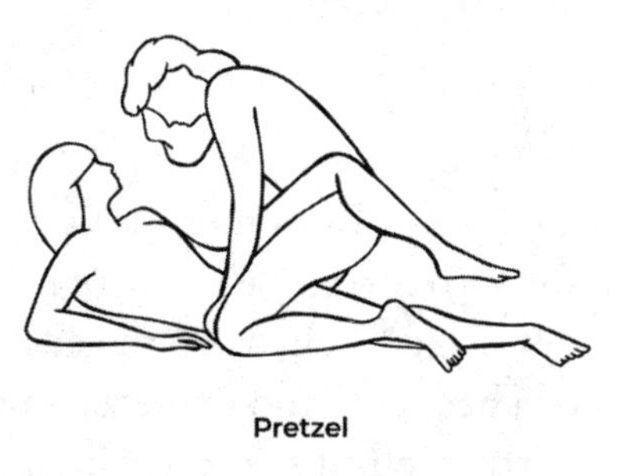

Pretzel

The Evolution: My advice here is to have the receiving partner angle their body so they're close to a firm surface, like a wall or a headboard. As the giving partner enters, the receiver can brace their hands, arms or feet against the surface to increase or decrease the intensity.

Both partners should thrust at the same time, with the receiver moving backward while the giver is moving forward, to allow for as much penetration as possible. Start off slow to get a matched rhythm and build speed once you're certain that you're both on the same page.

If the receiver keeps their legs closed, it can create a "tighter" sensation, which may feel particularly pleasurable for the penetrator. As a trade-off for deep insertion, spooning provides easy access to stimulate the receiver's chest, torso, and genitals with a hand or a toy.

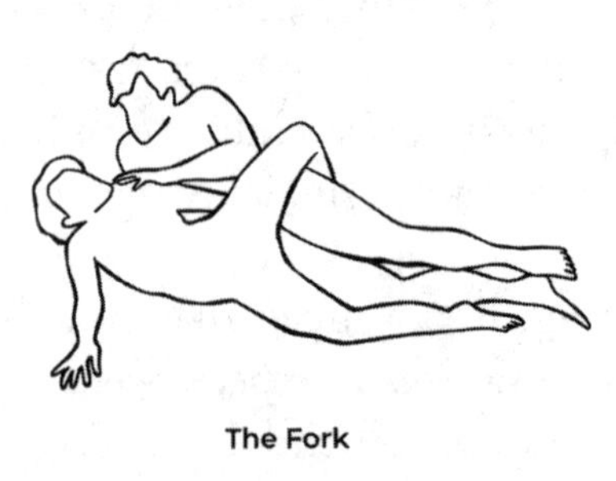
The Fork

A tweak on spooning is to have the receiver wrap their top leg back around the top of the giver's legs. This tweak, often called Forking, is far more optimal for G-area stimulation, while still providing plenty of access to the clitoris. The penetrator can also wrap their top leg around the receiver's body for extra skin-to-skin contact.

Another twist on this position (literally) is called the Pretzel. In this position, both partners lie down on their sides. The giver lifts the recipient's upper leg and straddles their lower leg, scooting closer until they have the right angle to enter. Then the giver folds over the receiver's torso, allowing them to wrap their arms around each other. Your limbs will be twisted, but you'll be face-to-face for eye contact and kissing.

Sitting

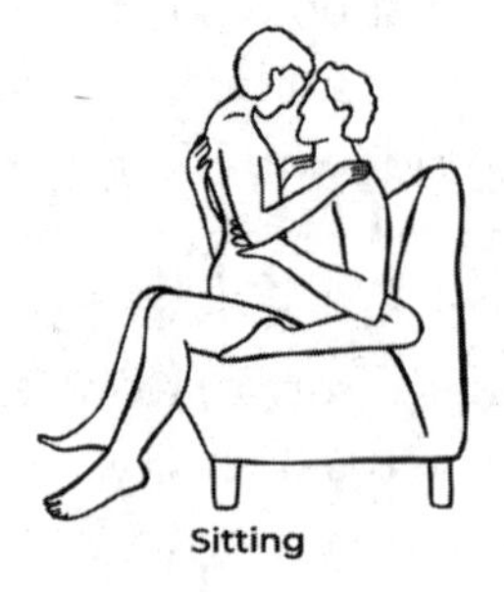
Sitting

The Basics: In its most straightforward form, the giving partner sits (on a chair, on the edge of a bed, etc.) and the receiving partner climbs into their lap, facing and straddling them.

The Pros: This is an incredibly versatile position. It can feel very intimate and romantic, with lots of eye contact, kissing, and even hugging during sex. It's also perfect for a hot and steamy session on a desk chair at work or even in the car.

This position is all about collaboration. It's up to you and your partner to create the vibe and overall experience that you're looking for. Plus, both partners have an opportunity to set the pace and the intensity, from a slow grind to an all-out bounce, slow and soulful, or vigorous and wild.

If the receiver is into it, they can lean back and create lots of erotic visuals while their partner holds on to their hips. Many receivers who enjoy cowgirl also like sitting for the same reasons—it's an opportunity to show off your body for your partner and to switch roles and be the one in the top position.

Your hands are pretty free in this position, and you can use them to explore your partner's body. Sitting also gives you a nice angle to nibble each other's necks, ears, nipples, and mouths.

The Cons: If you're on a soft surface, like a bed, leverage and balance can be a bit tricky. If at least one partner has their feet on the ground, you can get better leverage for deeper penetration and clitoral stimulation. But honestly, I can't think of many real downsides here. This is a great position.

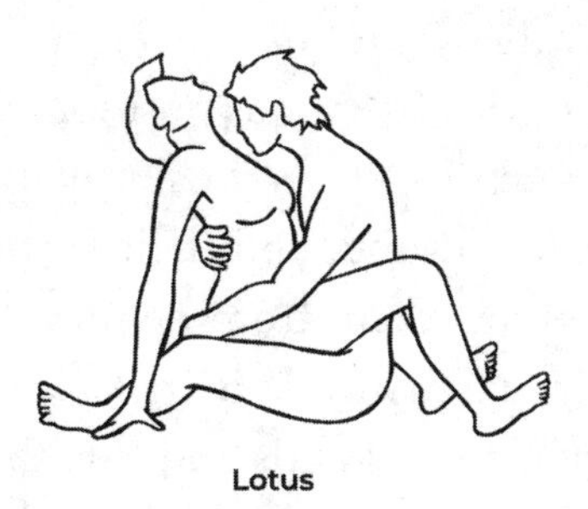

Lotus

The Evolution: You can turn sitting sex into a transcendent experience. Try breathing in unison and resting your foreheads against each other. In this position, you'll feel connected to your partner in every way: physically, mentally, emotionally, and spiritually. The intensity of the experience is so soulful, you'll want to slow it down, and drink it in. Who said that car sex couldn't be otherworldly?

If you prefer an up-and-down motion to rocking or grinding, have the giving partner sit with their legs stretched out in front of them. From there, the receiving partner straddles them, resting on their knees, and uses their thigh strength to perform a more hydraulic, up-and-down motion.

There are some variations to the sitting position. The first is the lotus, in which the giving partner sits with their legs crossed instead of flat on the floor. The receiving partner sits in their lap facing them, with their legs wrapped around the giver's torso. This position might feel amazing, or it may demand too much hip flexibility for you and your partner. Try it out, and make sure that the movement here is back-and-forth instead of up-and-down.

In the seated wheelbarrow position, the penetrating partner sits on the edge of the bed. Then the receiving partner faces away and positions themselves with their legs resting on the surface of the bed, their butt in their partner's lap, their torso resting on their partner's legs, and their hands on the ground in front of them. This position allows for deep penetration and isn't as strenuous as it sounds, but it does require the penetrating partner to do most of the work.

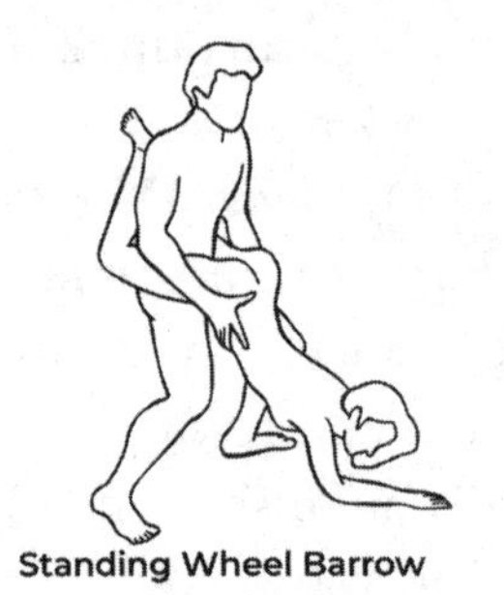
Standing Wheel Barrow

Side note: there is also a version of seated wheelbarrow called standing wheelbarrow. In this strenuous position, the recipient starts on all fours on the ground, and their partner enters them from behind. So, you're basically in a rear entry position. Then, the giver simultaneously stands and lifts their partner up by the thighs or the waist. The receiver wraps their legs back around their partners', while the giving partner supports their top half with their arms. Visually, it's like you're in position to do a wheelbarrow race at the county fair, but instead you're naked and having sex.

Slippery When Wet

Along with joining the mile high club and having sex in public, shower sex is on the top of many people's sexual bucket lists. I'm a big fan of masturbation in the shower, but I'm ambivalent about penetrative sex in a steamy, slippery stall. In fact, I used to be worried that I'd crack my skull until I found some solutions.

To me, shower sex seems to be one of those overrated, highly cinematic moments that looks so much better in the movies than it feels in real life. I have a friend who's an emergency room nurse, and I once asked her what sex acts sent most people to the hospital. She replied, "Foreign objects in the vagina and anus, and people with broken arms and noses and head wounds from falling in the shower." Damn.

If done safely, however, there are a lot of pros to shower sex that make it erotic, slippery fun. On a practical level, it is ideal for couples with roommates or kids. The sound of running water can drown out the moans, and the bathroom is already known to be a private space.

The shower is also the preferred place to try golden showers (peeing on each other) with no mopping up afterward, and shower sex is mess-free in general. Sweat and all other bodily fluids simply wash right down the drain.

As an added plus, a lot of people want to know how to make sure their partners are clean before sex. Shower sex is the answer. Get in there and give each other a good scrubbing, and you can kill two birds with one stone. Or shower together after sex for efficiency's sake, and see if you find yourselves going for round number two.

Here are a few tips to make shower sex as fun and safe as possible:

- **Take a strong position.** For the best balance, try a standing rear entry position. The receiving partner stands in front of the other, facing away and hinged forward at the hips. The giving partner stands behind them and enters from the rear. Depending on the size of the shower, the receiving partner can place their hands on their own shins or on the wall for extra support. Just make sure that the floor is not too slippery! You can buy an inexpensive shower mat for added security and confidence.
- **An even safer position:** If there's enough room, partners can do any version of the sitting position while the hot water rains down over your skin. (A bathmat in this position is not recommended.)
- **Give good shower head.** Does the shower have a detachable shower head? If so, you are #blessed to have a handy sex toy to play with. Many vulva owners have their first orgasm with a shower head or while letting running faucet water stream over their clitoris. Use it as part of good clean shower fun, either alone or with a partner.
- **Get handsy.** A small shower might not be the best place for penetrative sex, but it can still work well for hand and oral play. If you're using your hands, start with some hot mutual masturbation. If you opt for oral, take turns getting down on your knees. Don't try sitting on the edge of the tub to receive oral, though. It's too dangerous!
- **Use lube.** Lube is required, even in the shower. I know you're already wet from water, but it actually rinses

away your natural lubrication. And using soap as lube can be counterintuitively drying and potentially irritating. So, choose a silicone-based lube for the shower that lasts longer and won't just wash away like water-based lube.

- **Don't forget toys.** So many of today's sex toys are waterproof. Some dildos even have suction cups that you can adhere to the shower wall for easy play and accessibility. Just don't leave them there for your kids or roommates to find later! And the ease of cleanup is genius, whether you're using a vibrator, a dildo, or an anal plug.

Some people approach sex positions as if they're checking items off a list. But the real reasons to build our knowledge of sex positions are to expand our palette of sexual expression and to learn about ourselves so that we know exactly what we want and need to express. Then we can use that broad palette to approach partnered sex with intention. To feel experimental. To feel playful. To feel seen. To feel intimate.

Plus, we all get bored doing the same things over and over. We naturally crave variety to stoke our arousal. Trying a new position together can enhance intimacy with your partner.

Intimacy can take many forms, though, and next, we'll explore it in the realm that for many people is the most intriguing and elusive sex act...anal sex.

8

Get Ready, Willing, and Anal:

All Things Anal Play

I've noticed something over the past few years: anal sex is having a moment. I'm not sure if it's because anal has become so ubiquitous in porn, if it's because people are liberating themselves from what is basically the last frontier of sexual taboos, or if it's a combination of both.

In popular culture, we've seen anal sex go from something that was talked about with shock and horror just a couple of decades ago to something that is now pretty much mainstream. And the number of people trying it out reflects this. Between thirty and forty percent of heterosexuals have had anal sex at least once. (Frustratingly, because of lack of research, we don't have numbers for LGBTQ people.) And between ten and fifteen percent of heterosexual couples are having it regularly.

From where I sit, it's clear that close to a hundred percent of people are fascinated by anal sex. People ask me about it more than just about anything else. But even some of the most anal-curious people out there still have some hang-ups that are holding them back from giving it a go. Others have had a bad experience and are hesitant to try it again.

I get it. It took me many, many years to get comfortable with the idea of anal, but it is a unique and often intense form of pleasure. And there are other forms of anal play that don't involve insertion. There's plenty of fun to be had with toys, fingers, and analingus (also known as "rimming"), which is oral sex for the booty. There is no need to progress to penetration to experience anal pleasure—unless you want to.

Whether you're interested in light stimulation or full penetration, I have found that when approached with collaboration, consent, communication, and preparation, it can be an erotic, incredibly hot experience for all parties involved.

I hope that at the very least, you'll read this chapter with an open mind. If mental hang-ups are keeping you from trying anal, we'll work through some common myths and hopefully shift your mindset. If you've had a bad experience in the past, it's likely that you weren't fully prepared. Using the tips in this chapter, you may end up enjoying it this time around.

If you're already having anal regularly, I expect you already know that it can be a powerful source of pleasure that can also help build intimacy, exploration, liberation, and a meaningful sense of trust with yourself or with a partner. Whether you're already an expert in anal, consider yourself anal curious, or are dead set against it, I hope that this chapter helps you see this sex act in a new light while providing practical tips to make it safe, enjoyable, and fun.

Anal Myths and Anal Pleasure

First, let's clear up some myths around anal sex. Through fearmongering and even legal tactics, we have been conditioned to feel apprehensive about this very common sex act. Unfortunately, these myths are pervasive, leading many of us to avoid stimulating the booty at all costs and feeling like there's something wrong with us if we want to.

To this day, many heterosexual penis owners worry that wanting to be on the receiving end of anal means that deep down they must want to be with another penis owner, and are therefore gay. Remember that participating in a sex act doesn't define your sexual orientation. Plus, not all gay penis owners even enjoy anal sex, although they have definitely played a big role in making it more mainstream.

Many people are concerned that anal is dirty, shameful, and wrong. Even those that have gotten past all this are afraid that it will hurt or that their partner will be completely turned off if they suggest trying it out. Many people also believe that it's gross to get pleasure from a body part that's associated with waste.

This all comes down to nothing more than fear and shame. Anal sex is a breeding ground for shame more than almost any other sex act since it has been seen as forbidden for so long. Like oral sex, anal is still technically illegal in some states, although a Supreme Court ruling made it impossible to enforce these laws.

First of all, the laws against anal sex were created in order to discriminate against LGBTQ people. They are hateful and have nothing to do with the sex act itself. You are also not dirty for wanting to utilize this multipurpose body part for pleasure. Our bodies rid themselves of waste all the time through our sweat glands, our urine, and even our breath. The booty is no different, really.

I'd go as far as to argue that the anus was built for pleasure. The external anal sphincter, a ring of muscles that make it possible for the anus to open and close, is one of the most sensitive parts of the human body, with one the densest collections of nerve endings. When done correctly—slowly, with lots of preparation and breathing and plenty of lube—anal sex is not meant to be painful. Instead, all of those nerve endings can make anal stimulation feel really, really good.

Perhaps the best part is that we all have an anus. This makes anal the great equalizer of sex. Anal sex can also make both penis and vulva owners orgasm in new and different ways. In both cases, it may lead to deep internal orgasms. Imagine intense waves of pleasure that start deep inside your body and radiate out through the rest of your being. Yes, please.

In general, I find that penis owners are particularly curious about anal sex. For most cisgender heterosexual penis owners, their interest in anal is about them penetrating their partner. It's only been over the last few years that they have started to feel comfortable inquiring about or entertaining the idea of being penetrated themselves.

"Pegging" is a term that is commonly used to describe when a vulva owner penetrates their penis-owning partner with a strap-on or a dildo, although anyone with an anus can enjoy pegging. This still isn't widespread and certainly not something that most heterosexual penis owners talk about out loud (not yet). But it can also be extremely pleasurable. For the vulva owner, it can feel incredible empowering to be the one in charge.

Even among gay men, there is some stigma and shame around being on the receiving end of anal. It can be seen as "weak" or "feminine," which are not the same thing, and certainly not insults, thank you very much.

All I can say is that if I had a prostate, I would definitely want to see how it feels to have it stimulated. Once they try it, many penis owners of all sexual orientations appear to enjoy anal sex. Why? Because it feels amazing. Those sensations and the pleasure they experience say nothing about their sexual orientation. They simply tell you about your nerve endings. When stimulated correctly, nerve endings equal pleasure.

In penis owners, anal sex can lead to orgasm by stimulating the prostate, a gland that secretes fluid that nourishes and protects sperm. During ejaculation, the prostate squeezes this fluid into the urethra. It combines with sperm and fluid from another gland called the seminal vesicle to create semen, which is expelled from the body during ejaculation. This is your typical penile orgasm.

But when the prostate itself is stimulated, either by stroking it with a finger or a toy or anal sex, it can lead to a powerful orgasm that is more of an internal, full-bodied experience. It feels so good because there are so many nerve endings in the prostate. Plus, there is a shorter refractory period with a prostate orgasm than a penile orgasm.

Like all sex acts, though, enjoying anal isn't just about the pleasurable physical sensations. For some penis owners, it is a huge relief to not have to run the show during sex. For others, it's a fun way to play around with power dynamics and polarity. It's also a unique experience to be on the receiving end of something so vulnerable. Many penis owners find it to be very emotional for them, in a good way.

As well as being a sensitive area, the anus is a vulnerable one, regardless of your genitals. Anal play is not just a sex act. It can feel like a trust exercise and gift of total acceptance. To put your entire body into your partner's hands and to do it with an open heart and complete desire is a powerful act of surrender and intimacy.

It can be especially empowering for penis owners who experience erection difficulties to explore anal penetration. Remember, you don't need to have an erection to orgasm from anal sex! This gives anyone who can't have a traditional penile orgasm or is practicing semen retention to experience orgasm.

Vulva owners do not have a prostate gland, but their anuses were built for pleasure, too. Like penis owners, many of them shy away from anal play because of shame and/or because they feel pressured into it, like they "should" do it for their partner's pleasure and not their own. They may be especially hesitant if they tried anal in the past and it wasn't done correctly. Either their partner slipped it in by mistake or they did it too quickly without lube or proper warmup. In that case, it definitely can be painful, but it doesn't have to be that way.

When done properly, anal can be incredibly pleasurable for vulva owners. The vagina and rectum are separated by a single wall of muscle and share nerves, which is one of the reasons why anal can feel so pleasurable. The clitoral legs also extend all the way back to the anus, and there are shared nerves between the anterior wall of the rectum and the vagina. Anal sex stimulates all of these areas at once, leading to incredibly powerful orgasms (or just incredibly pleasurable sensations).

Sounds pretty good, right?

I know, I know. You're worried about poop, smells, the mess...all of it. I won't lie to you. Poop might happen. Smells might happen. Mess might happen. It's okay. All bodies poop and smell and secrete liquids. Sex is messy, just like life! Once we accept that, we'll be able to settle into less anxiety and more pleasure. I recommend investing in some gear to help manage the mess, including waterproof blankets, nitrile gloves, towels, and wipes.

My goal is to rebrand anal sex as a profoundly intimate and enjoyable sex act, not a taboo or something to be ashamed of or something that one partner "owes" to the other. With all of that said, anal sex does require a bit more attention to hygiene, a bit more prep, and a bit more lube than most other sex acts. So, now that I hopefully piqued your interest, let's make this exciting sex act as safe and stress-free as possible.

So Safe and So Clean

Many people worry that anal is dirty or dangerous because of the potential spread of bacteria from fecal matter. To lower those chances of spreading bacteria, the receiving partner or partners should ideally empty their bowels thirty to sixty minutes before anal play. It's not a requirement, but if it makes you feel more comfortable, you can also use an enema as part of your prep process. Be careful, though. The delicate skin around the anal opening can easily tear and can cause damage. This is obviously painful, plus it can lead to the spread of STIs if bacteria get into those tears.

If you choose to do an enema, buy one that comes pre-filled with enema fluid or an enema bulb made of silicone so you can fill it with warm distilled water at home. If you choose a pre-filled enema, I recommend that you empty out whatever solution it comes with and fill it with warm water. Then wash the outside of the anus with soap and water. That should do the trick.

But you know your body best. How we process waste varies from person to person based on our own digestive systems, our diets, and so on. Some people like to adjust their diet to eat small, light meals the day before they are planning to be on the receiving end of anal. There's no one way to prepare for anal, in part because no two anuses or rectums—or digestive systems—are exactly the same.

The next step is to wash your hands and trim your nails to avoid tearing. Thoroughly washing your hands before and after any and all anal play will prevent the spread of germs, and no one wants wolverine claws exploring their anal cavity.

If you have long nails and want to keep them that way, here's a great tip—place a cotton ball at the end of each nail and then put gloves on, securing the cotton balls in place. Voila—manicure maintained, anal canal protected.

Speaking of gloves, they're always a good idea for anal play so you don't have to run to the sink to wash your hands over and over. It helps prevent contamination and interruptions. Well-fitting latex gloves work well. If you're sensitive to latex, look for latex-free nitrile gloves.

The absolute best way to avoid tearing (and make anal a lot more pleasurable) is to use a lot (and I mean a *lot*) of lube. This goes for any type of anal penetration or insertion, including with a finger or a toy. Lube is the hero of anal sex. It is a nonnegotiable. The anus does not self-lubricate, so I can pretty much guarantee that attempting any type of anal penetration without a lot of lube will be painful and chafe the anus. If you think you're using enough lube, double it. Seriously.

The best type of lube for anal is silicone based. It lasts the longest so you don't have to reapply as often as you do with a water-based lubricant. Keep in mind that silicone lube can degrade silicone toys, so if you're using one of those, choose a water-based lube and reapply often. Definitely avoid oil-based lubricants, which can cause tears in condoms.

It's also important to avoid using numbing creams during anal. The anus is sensitive. Being even a little bit numb increases the chances of injury. Plus, it blunts the pleasurable sensations. Who needs that?

The final way to avoid infection is to follow this rule—no double-dipping! It's even more important for anal play than it is for chips and dip. If a penis or finger or toy makes contact with an anus and then makes contact with a vulva or a mouth, the spread of bacteria and infections is quite likely. Of course, this is true during solo anal play, too.

After any type of anal play, wash up thoroughly with soap and water. If you're playing with a partner, it can be fun to shower together. Then you're free to move on to any other sex act that you like.

It's important to note that condoms are especially important during anal because of the increased risk of infection due to tearing. Dental dams are highly suggested during analingus. It's also best to only engage in anal play when you and your partner are both sober and clearheaded. It has become a trend for people to take certain drugs beforehand to help them relax, but this can lead to increased risks. When you're under the influence, you may not be as attuned to your own sensations or cues from your partner, which can cause you to go too fast too soon. It's important to relax, but it's just as important to remain embodied and present. As you get more comfortable, you will be able to do both.

Anal Training

You're clean and prepped, but I'm sorry to say that you're still not ready to jump right into anal penetration. When it comes to anal, it's more important than ever to go slow. It will probably take some time to train your body and your mind to get used to having something inside of this very private and intimate area.

We tend to clench our sphincter muscles when we are even the slightest bit tense or anxious, and if you try to go from zero to anal, you're probably going to tense up. This will make penetration painful instead of pleasurable—something we definitely want to avoid. These muscles are also typically tight, even if you're not clenching. Just like you'd warm up and go slowly before attempting a full split, you want to make sure your sphincter muscles are strong and pliable.

It's just as important to get mentally comfortable with anal stimulation, especially if you're still working through any shame blocks. I strongly recommend that you engage in at least a few solo prep sessions to get mentally and physically ready before playing with a partner. It's best to spend about four to six weeks preparing alone.

In addition to the above reasons, starting your anal play alone will allow you to tune in and get to know which kinds of sensations you like and which ones you don't. Then you can communicate those preferences to a partner. It's also helpful to understand exactly what it's like to be penetrated. If and when the time comes to penetrate a partner, you'll have a clear idea of how it might feel and can make it as pleasurable as possible for both of you.

Even if you have no intention of trying anal with a partner, anal masturbation is a powerful way of giving yourself pleasure and getting to know your body. There is no reason to wait for someone else before experiencing all forms of pleasure.

The key for these solo sessions is to relax and go slow. Make sure that you're clean and that you have all the time and space you need. Do some breath work to calm your nervous system and create some erotic heat with yourself before digging in. Maybe light some candles and put on your favorite sexy music—whatever helps stoke your desire.

Start your session by generously exploring and stimulating your other erogenous zones with a hand or a toy or both. Remember to be incredibly mindful about choosing which hand will be exploring the anus and/or washing thoroughly in between anal stimulation and any other genital touching. This includes washing any toys. Yes, I'm repeating myself because it's that important.

As you're exploring, if you have a "traditional" orgasm first, that's great. You want to be as aroused as possible with lots of blood flow when heading into anal play. Penis owners, remember that you don't have to have an erection to enjoy anal play or even to have an orgasm!

When you're ready to go for the booty, take a minute to get in a comfortable position that gives you easy access. Lie on your back with your knees bent and your feet on the bed or with your knees splayed out to the side. Don't be afraid to use a mirror to find your anus. Seeing something with your eyes can help you tune in to the sensations you're feeling.

Now, breathe! Slowly and fully. This will help relax the nervous system and the sphincter muscles and promote blood flow. This is also the time to apply lube. Don't forget this important step.

From here, use the pad of a finger to circle around your sphincter muscles, remembering to relax and avoid clenching. Keep up that slow, deep breathing. Then try inserting a finger and see how that feels. You can keep it shallow at first and go deeper as you get more comfortable. Pay attention to what depth you prefer, what rhythm feels good, if some areas feel more sensitive than others, and when your muscles clench or relax.

For penis owners, can you find the prostate? The prostate gland is located inside and slightly down from the opening of the anus. How does it feel to stroke it? Does it feel better with gentle or firmer pressure? Harder or faster?

As you get more comfortable, you can insert another finger if you like. Don't hesitate to stimulate your genitals at the same time, either with your other hand or with a toy. This may take some practice, but the dual stimulation can feel ridiculously good.

Throughout your solo sessions, it's important to deploy your A-plus embodiment skills. You're exploring a part of your body that might be totally new to you, so it's crucial to pay really close attention so you avoid hurting yourself and can work through those mental blocks. It's possible that intrusive thoughts like "This is gross," or "This is scary," might pop up.

If you're really attuned, it's powerful to replace those thoughts with "This feels good," or "I am empowered to explore all aspects of my sexuality." Breathe through it. As you normalize this activity for yourself, those intrusive thoughts will fade away and you'll be able to access new levels of sexual pleasure in your own body.

If you don't have an orgasm, don't sweat it. It may take time. You explored a new aspect of your sexuality and likely learned something about yourself. Good job!

If you do have an anal orgasm, use those embodiment skills to glean valuable data. Try to notice if you can feel your sphincter muscles squeezing and clenching. Also, pay attention to what happens to your body *after* you orgasm. Does your anus relax or tighten back up? This is valuable information to have if you proceed to anal play with a partner. If you're someone who tightens, they might need to hold still during your anal orgasm and then release their toy, finger, or penis slowly and gently. And you should do the same thing during your solo sessions.

I strongly recommend spending the first few solo sessions exploring with just fingers. Then you're ready to move on...

Anal Toys

Despite the fact that anal is having a moment, anal toys haven't yet become mainstream. I think this will change in the near future. In the meantime, there are still some solid choices for you to explore, either during your solo sessions or with a partner. There are also anal training kits. These handy kits generally contain toys in three different sizes so you can work your way up.

I hope it goes without saying that you should never insert anything into your anus that wasn't made specifically for this purpose. Also, anything that you put in your anus must have a flared edge so it doesn't get lost in your body. Here are some of the most fun (and safe) options:

Butt Plugs

These are starter toys for many anal newbies. They're designed to be inserted into the anus and then left in place. Butt plugs stretch the sphincter muscles, helping your body adjust to being penetrated this way, and create a sensation of fullness that can feel really good.

You'll see butt plugs in a variety of shapes and sizes. The most important feature is that they're narrowest at the insertion point and get larger toward the flared base.

If you're a beginner, start with a butt plug that's on the smaller, shorter side and work your way up. As you begin to feel more comfortable and your sphincter muscles acclimate, you can look for wider girths, greater lengths, and even butt plugs that vibrate. Some people love the vibrating sensation in the anus, while for others it's too much.

Anal Beads

These are strings of five to ten silicone beads that are meant to be inserted into the anus. They start off very small at the insertion point and gradually grow longer. Unlike butt plugs, anal beads create more of a firework sensation than feelings of fullness.

The best way to use these is for you or your partner to insert a many of the beads as you like and then pull them out one at a time during orgasm. As your sphincter muscles clench against each bead, it emphasizes orgasmic muscle contractions.

Again, you don't want anything to get stuck in the anus. Always look for a loop or T-shaped handle at the end of your anal beads for easy, safe removal.

Anal Dildos

These are slightly more advanced, as they are made for full anal penetration and are often used for thrusting. They do not typically feature a tapered insertion point. This means that your muscles have to be ready to receive something that's bigger than the narrowed tip of a butt plug or beads.

You should still look for a flared base, however, so there is a very obvious, very secure way to get the dildo out. For this reason, I do not recommend using a garden variety dildo for anal penetration. It's worth springing for one that's made specifically for the anus.

Pegging Sets

These sets take anal dildos to the next level. More commonly called strap-ons, they feature a dildo that you can securely attach to a wearable harness. There are also "pegging panties," which are basically panties with a strap-on attached or a harness for you to attach your own.

Prostate Toys

There are many types of toys that are made specifically to stimulate the prostate. These include prostate massagers, anal vibrators, or curved butt plugs in the exact right shape to reach the prostate. Even better are vibrating prostate massagers and toys that stimulate externally and internally at the same time.

Communication and Consent

If and when you're ready to move on to exploring anal play with a partner, it's time to practice the communication skills we learned about earlier to broach this topic. I definitely don't recommend turning to your partner in bed and saying, "Hey, babe, want to try anal?" Remember the Three *T*s: Timing, Turf, and Tone. Use these to give yourself the best possible chance of having a productive conversation.

When it comes to talking to your partner about anal, the old adage applies: hope for the best, prepare for the worst, and take whatever comes. Hopefully, you!

For many couples, anal exploration is the ultimate trust builder. It requires a tremendous amount of collaboration, intimacy, and communication. The key to this conversation is to be clear about why this is something you want to explore *together.*

Maybe anal play is something that you've always wanted to try, and you trust this person enough to finally give it a go. Or maybe you feel that exploring in this area will help deepen your sexual connection. Telling your partner why this particular sex act appeals to you on an emotional level will lead to a more fruitful conversation.

Next, share any insights that you've gained from your solo explorations. What felt good about it? Why do you think this is something your partner would enjoy? Did you love using your fingers or toys? Letting them in on your process demonstrates a level of thoughtfulness around the activity.

Anal is still a very new sex act for most people, and it may take some time for your partner to get used to the idea. Partnered anal play only works when it is something that both people are enthusiastic about. It should never be something that one partner does just to please the other.

So, if your partner's initial reaction is a no or not yet, try to receive that response with grace. Focus on the positives of your existing sexual connection, and know that you may have to wait a bit for them to warm up to the idea. Or it might be something that they never come around to. In this case, you can continue exploring on your own and eventually decide how important partnered anal is to you.

If, on the other hand, your partner is into it, congratulations! But wait—the conversation isn't over yet. There are many different types of anal play. Make sure you're clear on which activities you'd like to try together.

Maybe your partner is into a little finger stimulation but isn't comfortable with analingus or penetration. Or maybe one of you wants to penetrate the other but doesn't want to be penetrated—or vice versa. It's important to know all of this beforehand so that you can relax and enjoy in the moment.

It can be fun to turn this into a game—"Yes, No, Maybe—Booty Edition." You've already done a lot of exploring by yourself, but keep in mind that this might be totally foreign for them. Having a menu of anal play behaviors will give them a chance to consider each one and create clear boundaries in a playful way. Your list can include any and all butt-centric activities, such as:

- Spanking
- Butt biting
- Giving/receiving anal massage
- Giving/receiving analingus/rimming
- Anal sex: being penetrated with a finger/penis/dildo
- Anal sex: you do the penetrating with a finger/penis/dildo

Another nice way to normalize anal sex for newbies is to watch ethical porn together that depicts anal in a positive, realistic way.

It can be especially helpful if it features a couple with genitals that match yours (a vulva owner with a penis owner, a penis owner with a penis owner, or a vulva owner with a vulva owner).

Finally, prepare to communicate often during the act itself. Anal play can be amazing, but the sensations involved are new and can at times be uncomfortable or even painful if you go too fast. If you're not sure if you're going slow enough, err on the side of caution and slow down even more. Consistently check in with each other to make sure that everything feels good, and stay connected to your partner's reactions, body language, and verbal cues throughout.

Establishing a safe word beforehand is also a great idea. This is a word that you agree to say in the moment if you want to stop. Then if either of you bumps up against a sensation that suddenly feels painful, you say the safe word and your partner knows to immediately halt whatever they're doing. If you're well prepared and go slow, you probably won't experience any sudden pain, but it's a nice guardrail to have, just in case.

A safe word system that's easy to remember is the traffic light: green, yellow, red. Obviously, green means keep going, yellow means slow down or proceed with caution, and red means stop. This can be helpful during all sex acts, not just anal.

Now, you are finally ready for the act itself! Let's get to it.

Partnered Anal Sex

The most important things to have for a safe and sexy anal sex experience as a couple are trust, communication, and relaxation (and lube, of course). Remember the mind-booty connection. As you breathe deeply and your mind eases, so will your sphincter muscles. When you're in an open, calm, and trusting state, it's far easier to let go and enjoy all the amazing sensations your booty has in store.

Just like when you prepped for anal masturbation, I recommend doing some whole-body relaxation exercises leading up to anal sex with your partner. Do some breathing exercises, take a bath, take turns giving each other a massage...any tactic that *you* love to help you release tension and get into your body.

You also might want to throw a towel down on the bed in case of any mess. It's normal. It happens. And this way, you don't have to worry about ruining your nice clean sheets.

Once you're ready, don't skimp on foreplay. You want to be as aroused as possible so that your muscles are relaxed and your blood is flowing. Familiar sex acts are totally welcome here and can be a nice gateway to anal play.

Anal Massage/Fingering

As an intro-level anal play activity, anal massage is usually the thing that most booty-curious folks try first.

To try anal massage on your partner, begin stroking their anus gently, drawing small circles around it with your finger. Next, rub the opening of their anus with one finger. Check in with them to see how that feels, and pay attention to your partner's sounds and body language. Are they moaning in pleasure? Or are they holding their breath and tensing up? Anal play is vulnerable, so stay communicative in the moment.

If you get the go-ahead, slowly progress from anal massage to fingering. Start with inserting one finger up to the knuckle. If your partner is into it, work your way up to two fingers or more, going as deeply as they like. Since you already explored this on your own, you can use the same steps to coach your partner to perform an anal massage and fingering on you, too.

Prostate Play

If your partner is a penis owner, now you can try to use your finger to stimulate their prostate. This can be as elusive and intimidating for vulva owners as finding the G-area is for penis owners. But it doesn't have to be that way. Try to relax and have fun with it.

Start by gradually pushing your longest finger all the way into the anus. The prostate gland is located inside and slightly down from the opening of the anus. You're trying to feel a firm gland that's about the size of a walnut. Remember that it will be easier to feel if your partner is already aroused.

Once you locate the prostate, gently stroke it. The prostate likes gradual stimulation. While you're stroking the prostate, you can place your thumb on the perineum and rub gently there, too. This allows you to stimulate the prostate both internally and externally. Side note—if your partner isn't into the idea of inserting anything into their anus, you can still stimulate the prostate by applying pressure to the perineum externally. You can also start here and work your way up.

After a while, you can try using slightly firmer pressure and see how your partner responds. Do they like circular movements, up-and-down, or side to side? Once your partner seems very aroused, continue to use repetitive, consistent movements. This can, and often does, lead to orgasm.

A-Spot Stimulation

If your partner is a vulva owner, you can try to find the anterior fornix or "A-spot," instead. There is actually some controversy over whether the G-area and the A-spot are just the back of the clitoris itself, which reaches around the vagina and urethra. Some experts believe that many vulva owners have a G-area that's located a bit deeper inside than others, and that's actually what we call the A-spot. Personally, I believe the G-area is a cluster involving clitoral nerves and other erogenous zones inside the body. Bottom line: anal play is a good way to reach this spot, and it can lead to powerful orgasms.

To stimulate this area, gradually insert a finger as deep in the anus as is comfortable. Curve it slightly toward their stomach, where the G-area is located. One or two inches inward from there is the so-called A-spot. You won't be able to feel the

A-Spot. It's an area inside the vaginal canal that's filled with nerve endings and can make the vulva owner very wet, very fast.

Sweep your finger up and down and from side to side using light pressure. If you feel moisture, that's a great sign. Check in with your partner to see how they like this area to be stroked.

A study actually tested how vulva owners responded to A-spot stimulation, and about forty percent had an orgasm, while almost eighty percent experienced increased lubrication. This means that more vulva owners will orgasm from anal stimulation than penetrative sex!

Analingus

Oral sex on the booty is a polarizing topic. Just as many people say that it's their favorite sex act as say that they would never do it in a million years.

Listen, it's your anus and/or your tongue. You should never feel any pressure to do anything that you don't want to do. But my personal opinion is that if everyone is clean and willing, why not try it? Our bodies are capable of experiencing so much pleasure. It seems like a waste not to explore all of the possibilities.

Of course, there are some times when you definitely want to skip this one. If anyone is experiencing gastrointestinal upset or has any type of sores, cuts, or hemorrhoids, save it for another time. Outside of these issues, analingus is a good way to get acclimated to anal stimulation. It's also a moment of radical acceptance that can be quite affirming for the receiver.

Another nice thing about analingus is that we all have an anus and we all have a tongue. It's a sex act that we can all give and receive with the same parts, regardless of our genitals. This means that if you've already received analingus, you know what feels good to you and can try those moves on your partner, and vice versa. This can make it extra hot and a nice point of connection.

To perform analingus on your partner, first have them get in position. They can lie down on their stomach with their booty perched up or on all fours for you to approach from behind.

If you'd rather approach from the front, they can lie on their back with a pillow underneath their hips. You can also try reverse face-sitting by lying on your back with them above you and facing away.

Now is a good time to get out the lube. In this case, why not try out some flavored lube? Then you're ready to proceed much like with oral sex. Lick around the anus in circles, half circles, or up and down, or push the tip of the tongue into the opening of the anus. Try different levels of pressure and see how they respond. You can tense your tongue to use just the tip or relax it to make it soft and utilize more of your whole tongue.

Don't be afraid to use your hands, too. In addition to spreading their flesh for more access, you can use a hand to reach around and stimulate their penis or vulva. This is a more advanced technique, for sure, but one that they'll probably love.

Along the way, pay attention to signals from your partner, including changes to the anus. When your partner gets more aroused, you might notice that the sphincter muscles soften and expand. That's a great sign that they're enjoying themselves.

After analingus is all said and done, take a moment to wash your hands and freshen your breath before moving on to any sex act of your choice, possibly including the showstopper of anal play...

Anal Penetration

First of all, there's no pressure to do it all, especially not right away. It's okay to stick with only anal rimming and/or a finger, and definitely go slow. I recommend rimming and massaging for a few sessions and then moving on to penetration, if and only if it feels right. This is an exploration, not a list of things you have to do.

If you do want to explore penetration, anal sex can involve a penis or a toy. Either way, make sure the receiver is highly turned on first. You want lots of deep breathing and blood flow to the genitals. You also want lots of lube—a fact that I can't emphasize enough.

Even with a lot of arousal and lube, penetration might need to be shallow at first. That's okay. Start with just the tip, go slow—even slower than you think you should—and hit the pause button if anything hurts. Add lube, change positions, or simply take five to breathe and check in.

When you become more experienced and want to move on to deeper penetration and thrusting, it might help to practice with smaller insertion devices (fingers, anal beads, etc.) to familiarize the anal canal with sensation. Once these smaller items feel good, you can go bigger, building up speed as you go.

As with any type of sex, there are various positions to try, each with their own pros and cons. Especially if you're a beginner on the receiving end of anal, make sure to use a position that will make you feel as comfortable and relaxed as possible. Here are a few good positions to experiment with:

Deep Spoon

For many anal rookies, this is often the most comfortable position. Try cuddling on your sides (spooning) with the penetrating partner as the "big spoon." In this position, it's easy for the receiving partner ("little spoon") to keep their anal muscles relaxed, which is key to this process. This is also a position that feels sweet and romantic, which can help ease any mental blocks that you may be working through.

Facedown

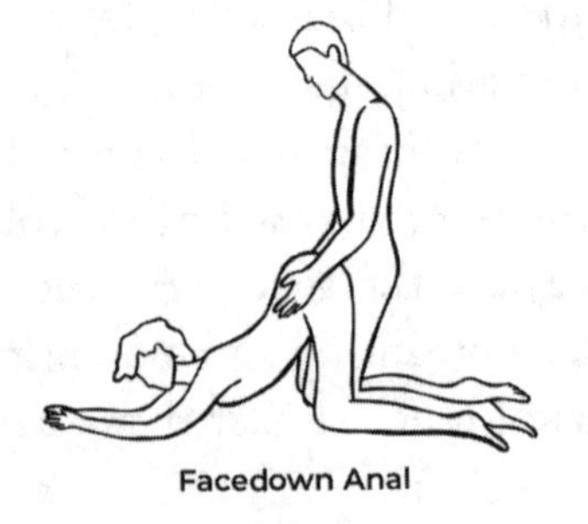

Facedown Anal

This is another fantastic option for beginners. The receiving partner lies facedown with their legs slightly apart. Or they can bend one leg at the knee and rest it on a pillow. From this position, the penetrating partner has lots of access and can easily brace their body weight with their hands.

There is no eye contact here, and it could potentially be triggering for those with lingering thoughts that anal is dirty or wrong. It's extra important to check in regularly and make sure that things are feeling good both physically and emotionally.

Missionary 2.0

This position is just like classic missionary, but with a sexy anal twist. Assume the standard position, and then have the receiving partner lift their legs and rest them on the giving partner's shoulders. This will allow for more access and lots of eye contact to enhance intimacy.

Standing Rear Entry

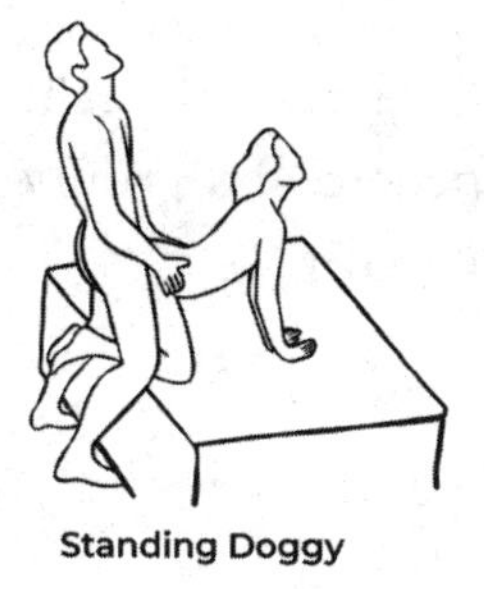

Standing Doggy

This position is exactly the same as your typical vaginal standing rear entry style but with a different entry point. The receiving partner braces their weight against something steady, like a wall or a piece of furniture, and the penetrating partner enters from behind. The penetrating partner can also use their free hand to stimulate the genitals, chest, or any other erogenous zone.

When you're done, put your towel in the laundry, wash your toys and hands with soap and water, and make sure to wash the outside of your anus (if you're the receiver) and the penis or toy (if you're the giver).

If you experience any irritation or a minor injury (it does happen), try taking a three- to five-day break, waiting until your stool is soft to re-engage. If you need to, try a stool softener or suppository that's made with cocoa butter to soothe the lining of the anal walls. After five days, you should start to feel better. If not, contact your healthcare provider, who can give you the care you need.

Speaking of care, there is one more important step that you should never skip...

Anal Aftercare

Aftercare is the way we check in and connect with our partners after any type of sex act. It should be a regular post-sex practice that enhances intimacy and helps us wind down after sex. Cuddling, pillow talk, showering together, kissing, giving each other a massage, or getting your partner a snack or a glass of water are all great examples of aftercare.

If you're not already, I encourage you to perform aftercare with intention after any and all sex acts. Aftercare can be especially important after anal, as it is inherently vulnerable. Aftercare ensures that everyone feels respected and grounded after whatever did or didn't just happen sexually.

For emotional aftercare, try:

- Deep breathing together. Close your eyes and ground yourselves with a few connected breaths.

- Cuddling. Spend time in each other's arms with an energy that's safe and soothing, rather than adventurous and erotic.

- Talking. Discuss what you liked and didn't like. This is a healthy practice after any sex act, but especially after anal, and particularly if it's new to either or both of you.

Exploring anal play is a way of growing in all of the Sex IQ pillars. When we are embodied, we can feel pleasure in a new and exciting area. When we are in good health, we know that our booties and minds are ready to engage in this way. With collaboration, this act can enhance our intimacy and connection with our partner. When we have self-knowledge, we can discern whether or not anal is something that we actually like. And when we accept ourselves, we can transform shame in this act into pride in our erotic range.

Anal play truly helps you get the most bang for your booty. Once you try it, you might discover that there is even more sexual pleasure available to you than you ever realized.

Now that you're in an adventurous mood, it's time to explore and play, and maybe—just maybe—get a little bit kinky.

9

Explore and Play:
An Accessible Guide to Kink

Years ago, when I started exploring my sexuality, I dated a guy who was much more experienced than I was in the world of kink. He knew I was intrigued, so he brought me to a sex dungeon—a facility that's set up for kinky play. This was a first for me. As we walked through the dungeon, I checked out all of the leather and whips and chains and flogs, and I have to admit it—I was a little bit turned on. And when he blindfolded me and I was able to surrender to him without knowing what was going to happen next, I was more than just a little turned on.

This is probably similar to what you imagine when I say the word "kink": edgy and kind of scary stuff like dungeons, whips, and chains. That is definitely one side of kink. But this is an area of sexuality that includes a wide spectrum of activities. There is an extreme end, but there's another end that's lighthearted and very accessible.

So, what is kink anyway? The technical definition of kink is anything sexual outside of conventional sex. This of course begs the question, what is conventional sex?

Take a minute now to close your eyes and imagine it. What do you think of when you picture conventional sex? For most people, it's a couple making out, falling onto the bed, engaging in some missionary-style sex, orgasming quickly, and falling asleep. Or something along those lines, anyway.

Do you engage in any sexual activities outside of what I just described? If so, then you might just be kinkier than you think.

Besides giving you plenty of ideas about how to dip your toe (or even your whole foot) into these waters, my goal in this chapter is to clear up a lot of misconceptions about kink and change the way you see it from something that's dark and taboo to playtime for adults. Think about it—as an adult, when do you really get a chance to let loose and have fun and explore? Kink is a way of merging your creativity with your eroticism. It's healthy, it's good for relationships, it can actually be very healing, and it is for everyone.

Kink and Your Sex IQ

Besides all of the other benefits, exploring your kinky side is a powerful way of growing all five of your Sex IQ pillars. This is where it finally all comes together!

All kinky activities, from talking dirty to spanking to role-playing, require you to be embodied and present. You'll be less likely to disassociate and go off into fantasyland in your mind while you're engaging with your partner in this intense way. This presence is good for your health, particularly your mental health. It allows you to start associating sex with play, connection, and a state of flow, which is healing.

In a state of flow, the past and future cease to exist in our minds. It also helps to ease anxiety and enhance focus. We're so deliciously caught up in the playful, hot, exciting thing we're doing that our worries tend to fall away.

Kink is also one of the most effective ways to collaborate and connect with your partner on a deep level. Some aspects of kink are basically forms of power play and polarity, particularly BDSM (bondage and discipline, domination and submission, and sadism and masochism). In all types of BDSM play, there is a consensual power imbalance. One partner is dominant, and the other is submissive. This is a great way to play around with polarity.

Collaboration is a big part of many other types of kinky play, too, like dirty talking and role-playing. Learning to collaborate in this way is great for relationships. So many long-term partners stop having fun together after a while, both in and outside of the bedroom. But couples that play together, stay together.

Kinky play also builds trust and improves communication. In order for kink to be fun and safe for everyone, excellent communication is a must. You need to be able to create clear boundaries and the limits of how you will interact and treat each other during playtime, just like you would in the day-to-day aspects of your relationship. These communication skills often spill over into other areas of relationships. Trust me, if you can negotiate a BDSM scene together, you can probably decide who's making dinner.

Earlier, we discussed core desires—or the feelings we most want to experience during sex. Uncovering these is a big part of our self-knowledge. Often, these core desires can be deeply experienced through kinky play. This type of play provides a palette for us to explore our feelings in a safe context, not just a socially acceptable one. Especially if you were ever told that your feelings were bad or wrong or invalid, this can be really healing. In this way, kink helps us grow in our culminating Sex IQ pillar—Self-Acceptance.

Kink Versus Fantasies and Fetishes

Before we move on and start learning about how to explore kink, I want to clear up some common misconceptions around kink, fetishes, and fantasies and how they relate to each other. Many people think that all three are basically the same thing, but they are actually all completely different.

We've already defined kink as any type of sex that isn't "conventional." It may help to think of fetishes and fantasies as sitting underneath the umbrella of kink, as they're both outside our culture's narrow definition of conventional sex.

A fantasy is simply anything that turns you on when you imagine it. You can fantasize about certain people, specific sex acts, you name it. Most of us have our go-to fantasies that we think about when we're masturbating or getting turned on. These can range from very simple images to complex scenarios and everything in between.

It's important to know that just because you fantasize about something, that doesn't necessarily mean that you actually want to experience it. Often, it's enough to think about this fantasy while masturbating or sometimes during partnered sex. It doesn't have to translate into real life.

For example, it's common to develop fantasies from things you see in porn that probably would never happen in real life. Or you might fantasize about having sex with your coworker or your neighbor, even though you would never actually do it, and you'd be mortified if anyone knew you thought about them while masturbating. You might not even find them attractive! A lot of people feel shame around this or feel guilty for fantasizing about other people when they're in a relationship, but this is completely normal and healthy.

However, there may also be times when you realize that you actually do want to experience something that you've been fantasizing about. It can be healthy and fun to explore your fantasies with a partner, as long as you communicate about it clearly and make sure that everything is safe and consensual.

Fetishes, however, are different from fantasies. Many people misuse the term fetish. They say, "Oh, I have a fetish for redheads" just because they once dated a redhead and still fantasize about how hot the sex was. In reality, a true fetish is defined as a requirement for arousal, not just something that turns you on. In other words, fetishists rarely get aroused without having a specific object or circumstance present.

There are many theories and assumptions, but we don't know exactly why some people develop fetishes and others do not. Like core desires, fetishes might be tied to childhood events, but also could be linked to other life experiences. Sometimes there's no clear link or explanation. Fortunately, you don't have to understand something to validate or respect it.

It can be difficult to have a fetish that puts conditions on your sexual arousal, and the research shows that they are not easy to undo. My advice for fetishists is to find ways to work with your fetish instead of trying to deny or change it. You can still have a healthy relationship with someone who does not share the fetish. It just takes a lot of open communication and compromise.

To make this work, try to gradually bring your partner into it and make them a part of the experience. For example, if you have a latex fetish, tell your partner how hot you think it would be to buy them a latex outfit. See how they like it, and then have a conversation about how and when you're going to incorporate the fetish into your sex life.

If, however, you think it would be really hot to see your partner in latex, but it's a "nice to have" instead of a must, that's a fantasy, not a fetish. And if you and your partner decide to incorporate a little latex into your sex life once in a while, that's not a fetish, either. It's some good old-fashioned kink—a fantasy brought to life.

Whether you're embarking on a fantasy, a fetish, or any other sort of kink, make sure to use your best communication skills to discuss it with your partner beforehand. You can use the Yes, No, Maybe list on page 127 to start this conversation. Set clear boundaries and agree to a safe word. Remember the traffic light system:

red, yellow, green. This works well here and can allow you to both relax and lean into the fun and excitement without any concerns about lines getting crossed. It's also especially important to be intentional about aftercare after kinky play with your partner.

Now, let's take a look at some of the most common forms of kink and exactly how (and why) you might want to partake in them.

Talk Dirty to Me

One of the best ways to incorporate your brain into your sexual experiences is through dirty talk. Despite its name, dirty talk doesn't have to be *dirty*. By definition, dirty talk is any words or sounds that increase arousal and sexual pleasure. Sure, it can be graphic or naughty or downright filthy, but it can also consist of a simple moan or a single word—*Yes, More, Harder, Deeper...*

If you're new to dirty talk and feel awkward or unsure about how to start, at first you can just make some noise. Practice moaning and groaning in pleasure during solo sex to get used to using your vocal cords when you're aroused. This will help you feel more comfortable doing the same thing with a partner. Added bonus: humming and moaning stimulate the vagus nerve, which is the "off" switch for stress. It makes sense then that many of us naturally moan during sex!

After you're gotten more comfortable making those pleasure-laced noises, you can start to get creative and use words. Slowly start to find your voice and say what's comfortable. No one expects you to sound like a porn star. You want your dirty talk to sound genuine and like you—or the sexy, kinky version of you.

An easy on-ramp to dirty talk is to say what you want or like. No flowery language needed. Just state it plainly. "I want you to play with my balls," or "I love it when you pin me down." You can also vocalize what you're feeling in the moment: "You feel so good inside me," or "I am so turned on right now." If the words come out as affirming and genuine, they will encourage your partner and excite you both.

Whenever you don't know what to say, you can just ask a question. It's sexy to hear, "Does that feel good?" Or, "Do you like that?" Plus, asking for feedback is a great way to enhance pleasure if you try to incorporate that feedback however you can.

A more advanced form of dirty talk is fantasy creation—describing activities to construct a particular fantasy or image in your partner's mind. These descriptions can be about what's going to happen later ("I can't wait to go down on you"), a previous sexual encounter that you both enjoyed ("I loved the way you tasted when I went down on you"), or a mutual fantasy ("Imagine how hot it would be if someone was watching me going down on you right now"). Fantasy creation can unlock a treasure trove of sexual energy and arousal, but check in with your partner to ensure they're enjoying the experience, too.

It's also fun and flirty to talk dirty over text, and many dirty talk newbies actually feel more comfortable with this. It can be less intimidating to type something to your partner than it is to say it to them. Another perk to sexting is that when you send sexy messages about what you're going to do and how good it's going to feel, you're priming yourself and your partner to be excited. This heightens arousal and desire. Plus, it'll be easier to say things in the moment that you've already said over text.

With sexting and dirty talk in general, the goal is to have a fun sexual experience with your partner. Don't be afraid to be silly and laugh. It doesn't always have to be serious and sultry. If you try it out and feel overwhelmed, stressed-out, or self-conscious to the point that you're not having fun, take a break. You can try again later or even decide that dirty talk just isn't for you. There are plenty of other fun things that you can try.

BDSM

When most people refer to BDSM, they're simply talking about sexual activity with defined power roles between partners. To a mild or extreme extent, one person is dominant, and the other person is submissive, or they might switch roles. BDSM can involve bondage (tying someone up or restricting their movement), sadism (getting pleasure out of inflicting pain), or masochism (getting pleasure out of experiencing pain). At its core, BDSM is a consensual power imbalance where someone is in control (the Dominant or Dom) and someone else has relinquished control (the Submissive or Sub).

It makes sense that people who haven't played around with this kink often don't understand why anyone would want to give their power away, especially during sex. But this isn't always the case. It can simply mean that one partner agrees to take a more passive and receptive role while the other takes control with a more assertive role.

This makes the roles during play very clear, and that clarity alone can be refreshing. On top of that, a sexual spark can be ignited when these dynamics create a contrast in energies. This is polarity in action, and it can play out in a variety of ways, ranging from subtle to very dramatic.

Many people naturally gravitate toward either a submissive or dominant role. Others like to switch and feel comfortable in either role, sometimes depending on the day or their mood. If you're not sure which one you're interested in trying, mine the contents of your fantasies and try to pick up on themes. In your fantasies are there any themes of restraint or of someone doing something to you? Those could be characteristics of a submissive stance.

Lots of people have a core erotic desire around being submissive during sex because elsewhere in life they have to be responsible, self-directed, and in charge—and it's usually been this way since childhood. Having someone else tell them what to do is a relief. Now *they* get to be directed and even bossed around, and this can feel incredibly liberating.

On the other hand, are there themes in your fantasies of you telling people what to do or issuing commands? Do you enjoy seeing other people squirm a little? Those are characteristics of a dominant side.

Lots of people have a core erotic desire around being dominant during sex because elsewhere in life they are lacking a sense of control or agency—and probably have since childhood. Calling the shots during sex feels empowering. Now *they* get to be the boss and enforce a sense of discipline.

Once your roles are established, decide beforehand how far you're going to take these roles. Is the dominant partner simply going to lead during sex, or are they taking a more aggressive stance? Will you establish power through communication (using a special name like "Daddy," or having the dominant partner use dirty talk through degradation, praise, or a combination of both)? Power play doesn't have to involve anything physical, and it doesn't even have to involve sex. It can add an exciting dimension to your sex life using just words.

If you do want to take it a step further, decide if the submissive partner will have to follow rules, like they can only orgasm when the dominant partner says so. Will there be a punishment, like a nice spanking, if they don't follow the rules?

Also decide if the dominant partner is going to restrain the submissive or take away one or more of their senses. Wearing a blindfold heightens the other senses. Plus, it can be incredibly exciting to not know what's going to happen next. Restraints, like a scarf, handcuffs, leg spreader bars, or rope made for bondage put the dominant partner in complete physical control, which can be very exciting for both parties. Of course, it's important to make sure you are on the same page and establish limits, boundaries, and a safe word or signal beforehand.

Dominating Through Text

Some dom/sub couples play with these power dynamics in all areas of their relationship, while others keep it strictly within the sexual realm. One small way to take this outside of the bedroom is over text (with prior consent, of course).

As the dom, you might give your sub commands and instructions to masturbate at a certain time of the day, or set a rule that they cannot masturbate or can only tease themselves without orgasming until you give them permission to do so. Or you could instruct them on what to wear or eat to take better care of themselves. (Doms can be loving! Don't mistake dominating your partner for being cold or cruel. While being told what to eat or wear might be construed as abusive to some people, it can also be a part of a consensual dom/sub relationship.)

If you're into this, try, "I want you to tease yourself all day today," or "I'll be home in an hour. I want you naked and on the bed when I walk in," or "Put on the blue shirt I picked out for you for dinner tonight."

Depending on what they do, texting either your pleasure or displeasure will correct bad behavior and reinforce good behavior. Try, "Good girl. I'm going to go down on you for an hour tonight as a reward," or "Bad boy. You can't orgasm tonight," or "As a punishment, I'm going to tie you up and tease you later."

Another great way to establish your dominance over text is to use commands and questions as a form of call and response. For example, "Does baby girl deserve Daddy's attention?" Or "Did you follow all of the rules today, as I requested?" Or a simple, "Understand?" If they don't respond, a punishment might be in order...

As always, sexting isn't just about what you say, but how you say it. Before you get into your digital dom play, think about your tone. Using the third person is a great way to establish some credibility and dominance.

For some subs, it's more powerful to receive a text that says, "Daddy is going to punish you," than simply, "I am going to punish you." It's a subtle but hot difference. If your partner is into this, give it a go and see how the power dynamics shift.

Also, don't forget to check in with your sub via text with messages that are as nurturing as the others are dominating. It's important to balance the control aspects of BDSM with something that's loving and compassionate. Remember that subbing, even over text, can be incredibly vulnerable. Think of this as dominant sext aftercare.

Now that you have some tips on text domming, whip out your phone and send a sexy command. Consider that an order!

For those who are into BDSM, here are a few ways to take it up a notch:

CNC (Consensual Non-Consent)

This is an admittedly controversial kink around pretend forced sex that is fully consented to beforehand. In other words, one partner has agreed to have pretend forced sex, and both partners are clear on the limits around touch, words, intensity, and other important aspects of play.

Fantasies about CNC, or "rape fantasies," are extremely common among vulva owners, but there's a lot of shame and misunderstanding around it. No, it does not mean that they want to be raped. Sometimes, the person has experienced a sexual assault and is attempting to work through it with this fantasy. This can be confusing and a source of shame for assault victims, but it is very common. The healthy way to do this is to work with a trauma informed therapist.

Another common reason for this fantasy is that vulva owners have been conditioned to feel shame and guilt around sex, particularly for wanting or initiating sex. It's freeing to be exonerated of all responsibility by being "forced" into it. For many, the idea that someone wants them so badly that they have to use force is really hot. It makes them feel irresistible, like their partners desire and crave them so much they can't help but force sex with them.

Of course, CNC requires a lot of trust and excellent communication. Exploring this particular kink in a way that's emotionally safe for everyone starts with a conversation. Decide in advance how you'd like the scenario to play out and anything that's off-limits. And it's especially important to have a safe word here that isn't "no" or anything else the partner may say as part of the fantasy in case something happens in the moment that makes them truly uncomfortable and they want to slow down or stop. If this happens, saying no or stop might be misinterpreted as part of the act. If done safely and it is truly consensual, this kink can be very exciting for a lot of people.

Pain Play

Whether it's a little love bite or a full-fledged whipping, inflicting or experiencing some level of physical pain is another popular kink—and for good reason. The pain processing center of your brain is incredibly close to your pleasure processing center, and they are in constant conversation. This leads your pleasure and pain centers to light up simultaneously during some stimulating events, such as eating spicy foods or having rough sex. Pain also increases the heart rate and blood flow, two essential ingredients of arousal.

Your body also releases many of the same chemicals when you are in pain and when you are turned on. This often leads pain play practitioners to experience a floaty or high feeling from the endorphins that flood the system when they experience pain.

It can be compared to a runner's high. A little consensual pain during sex also forces presence. It's hard to be stressed about work when your rear is stinging from a spank and your whole body is aroused.

Hence the phrase "It hurts so good."

This all leads pain play to be extremely common and arousing. You don't have to be a full-on masochist to enjoy this. Studies have shown that approximately sixty percent of vulva owners enjoy rough sex, which usually involves at least a little bit of pain. Again, consent is especially important here and needs to be clear, coherent, willing, and ongoing.

For beginners, temperature play can be a good way to explore the world of pain. It adds a little bit of shock to sex without being too painful. Try sucking ice before giving oral or rubbing a piece of ice up and down your partner's torso or along their inner thighs. If you're into heat, try body-safe candles (not regular candles, which can burn). With these candles, you can safely drip the wax onto your partner's body without causing burns because these candles are designed to melt at a lower temperature. Some candles are made of wax that turns into massage oil when it melts and you can then use it to rub each other down. Give them a massage, or simply drizzle it onto their skin to heighten arousal.

Another popular on-ramp for pain play is spanking or impact play. If you're new to this, try rubbing your partner's butt first to send the signal that you're about to begin. When you're ready, pull back, and bring the palm of your hand down on one of their butt cheeks. Start with a decisive spank, gauge how they react, and if they want it, you can work your way up to more intense contact.

As you and your partner get more comfortable with spanking, you can work in props, like a paddle or a hairbrush. If it has a flat, hard surface and can be held in your hand, it can be used to spank someone's butt.

Flogging and whipping are considered the next level up on pain play. Each of these props is available in a variety of materials. Floggers are made of strands of material, usually leather, that are held in place by a handle and can be used on multiple parts of the body. Just be sure to avoid the stomach and sides of the body. We don't want to flog anyone's internal organs.

Drawing blood is a real possibility depending on what you're using and how much force is being used. Caution is a must. For both flogging and whipping, my top recommendation is to learn from a professional. There's a technique to both, and while pain can definitely be pleasurable, if done improperly, it can be very unpleasant and even cause injury.

Finally, one of the most extreme forms of pain play is erotic asphyxiation or breath play (aka choking). The first and most important thing I want to say about it is that it's dangerous. It can cause you to lose consciousness and has caused a significant number of accidental deaths. Okay, with that said, many people enjoy choking or the sensation of having someone's hand on their throat. Cutting off oxygen, however briefly, can make a person feel lightheaded and dizzy, which can cause a rush. When the pressure is released and blood and oxygen resume their flow, there's a second rush, caused by the release of dopamine, serotonin, and endorphins. This second rush can also include a psychological component. You just trusted this person to choke you, which was pretty intense. And now all of these feel-good chemicals make you feel thankful and even euphoric.

To explore this kink safely, take some time first to learn about the anatomy of the neck, head, and chest. This goes for both the giver and receiver. Whatever you do, don't press directly on anyone's trachea (the wind pipe). Safer breath play can involve putting pressure on either side of the trachea. Incremental increases will help you avoid injury, so if you're intrigued, go slow—slower than you think you should. It's important to be extra careful. And it's worth repeating that whatever you do, never do it without clear consent.

Role-playing

We're all familiar with the cliché fantasy of a sexy French maid or a pizza delivery guy. Role-playing, or pretending to be someone else or yourself in an unusual scenario or environment can be this simple, or it can be extremely complex with full-on costumes, character development, and dialogue. I find this kink to be an especially playful and fun one for long-term partners to explore. You get to feel like you're having sex with someone new while remaining in the safe container of a committed relationship.

I once spoke to a couple of penis owners who had been together for ten years and felt that their sex life had grown a bit stale. I suggested that they each show up at a bar presenting as an alter ego. I call this a sexy stranger role-play experience. They flirted and had a drink at the bar and talked as if they were strangers who were getting to know each other for the first time. I was thrilled when they got back to me and said that they'd had the hottest sex of their lives later that night.

Sometimes all it takes is a wig. If you're used to having sex with a brunette, it can be thrilling to suddenly be with a blonde. It can also be incredibly liberating and sexy to explore another side of yourself through an alter ego or character. It's a fun way to see yourself and/or your partner in a new light. The point here is that role-playing doesn't have be intimidating. Just adding a new element like a wig might be all you need in the moment to make your sex feel varied and hot.

Role-playing Ideas

Of course, your favorite role-play scenario may harken back to your core desire. For example, if you want to feel a little naughty or transgressive, you may want to role-play two people having an affair. Or, if you want to feel worshipped, you can role-play a celebrity and their biggest fan. Here are some fun ideas for role-playing. You can pick out the ones that appeal to you and compare notes with your partner:

1. Teacher/student
2. Bartender/customer
3. Doctor/patient
4. Delivery person/customer
5. Alien/person who is abducted by alien
6. Yoga instructor/student
7. Boss/employee
8. Librarian/bookworm
9. Forbidden lovers
10. Devil/angel
11. Celebrity/manager
12. Police/criminal
13. Firefighter/rescued person
14. Two virgins having sex for the first time
15. Tarzan/Jane
16. Barista/customer
17. Two people having an affair
18. Criminal/hostage
19. Housekeeper/maid/pool attendant
20. The last two people on earth
21. Lifeguard/victim
22. Canvasser/voter
23. Sex worker/client
24. Therapist/client
25. Masseuse/client
26. Two coworkers
27. Teacher/parent
28. Flight attendant/pilot

29. Sailor/captain
30. Actor/director
31. Two neighbors
32. Artist/muse
33. Celebrity/fan
34. Athlete/trainer
35. Porn star/director
36. Assistant/boss
37. Fairy-tale princess/prince
38. Scientist and creation
39. Pizza delivery person/customer
40. Hitchhiker/person giving them a ride
41. Soldier/drill sergeant
42. Waiter/customer
43. Two superheroes

Voyeurism/Exhibition

This is one of the most common forms of kink out there. Voyeurs fantasize about watching someone else have sex, masturbate, undress, or do anything else private that outsiders don't normally see. Exhibitionists are the opposite. They get a thrill from being watched in private.

If you're into this kink, it may mean that you like being a little transgressive. Many people get turned on by doing things that they "shouldn't" be doing. Some love the thrill of potentially being caught.

To start playing with voyeurism, you can watch your partner bathe, undress, or masturbate (with previously given consent, of course). It can also be fun to watch yourself have sex in front of a mirror. Some enjoy bringing a third person into the bedroom and watching their partner have sex with them.

If you want to explore exhibitionism, you can ask your partner to "secretly" watch you during a private moment. Touch yourself, or perform a dance for them. Or think about having sex outside. This can be somewhere relatively private like your backyard, or somewhere bolder like a camping trail or in a parked car.

Keep in mind that public sex or exposure is illegal, and passersby haven't consented to watching you. Limit this to a remote area. You can experience the thrill of potentially being caught without anyone actually seeing you. Always be respectful of others while playing.

Humiliation

If you don't enjoy this feeling, it may be hard to imagine why someone would be turned on from being humiliated. We all have core wounds, just like we all have core desires.

Sometimes, people turn to kink to help reframe a core wound. It allows them to revisit it with a sense of control and generate a different outcome. For example, someone who had a tumultuous childhood and grew up among chaos may now crave structure and dominance and find that being a sub is incredibly healing.

Here's a more extreme example: I know a wealthy and successful penis owner who is extremely powerful in his business. In many ways, he's the stereotypical alpha male. And his deepest erotic craving is to put on a diaper and have a dominatrix urinate on him.

With self-awareness, he realized that this stemmed from his core wounding of being bullied as a child. It was extremely traumatic, and he never really got over it. Now, no matter how much money he makes or how many times he gets written up in *Forbes*, that bullied kid is still inside of him.

When he's with his dominatrix with his diaper on, this man is replicating his core wounding. But this time, he's the one in charge. Although he's being dominated, he sought out the experience, which means that he is ultimately empowered to decide whether or not it happens and how it happens. By playing out his core wounding in this way, it no longer has the same control over him. In the confined, safe world of kink, he's working out his wounds, and in doing so, healing them. I think that's pretty awesome.

If you want to try this, you can start by having your partner talk down to you or force you to beg or grovel. Words that would be shocking in day-to-day life can be used in service of arousal. If you have a humiliation kink, it may turn you on to be a called things like a bitch, whore, servant, or pussy, or to be spoken to with extreme disrespect or derision. To take this further, you might want to put on a collar and be led by a leash or have a partner ejaculate in your face or even urinate or defecate on you.

Another common form of the humiliation kink is cuckolding, when one partner consensually "cheats" on their partner specifically to humiliate them. Often, the cheating partner then shares all of the details to further humiliate the cuckolded partner. Sometimes, they even watch, while the third-party brags about their ability to please the cuckold's partner.

If any of this speaks to you, no judgment, and try not to judge yourself, either. We don't choose our core desires. There is nothing shameful about accepting and owning them and choosing to transform them into erotic play. When you stop judging yourself, you're able to let go and work with your authentic turn-ons rather than fight against them.

A Kinky Community

If you're inspired to explore your kinky side, you may be wondering how to find someone to explore with. Maybe you have a partner who's down to indulge your kink with you. Or maybe you have a partner who's not interested, or you don't have a partner at all. As long as you're honest with your partner (if you have one), none of this should stop you from exploring on your own.

Of course, you can explore many of the kinks we've discussed during solo sex. Pain play works especially well here. The most important aspect of kink is that it helps you get to know yourself in an extremely intimate and vulnerable way. Once you accept this part of yourself, you can actively seek out people who know how to turn that self-awareness and self-acceptance into pleasure.

If you want to find someone to play with, you might be surprised by the number of thriving kinky communities out there. Underground networks that are kink-friendly range from online communities like FetLife to apps like Feeld.

It can also be fun to take an in-person class led by a dominatrix or other kink expert. Since you are practically guaranteed to meet people who are interested in the same kink activities that you are, this is a great way to network and meet potential playmates.

Or take a note from my history book and visit a sex dungeon to find your community. I know this might be intimidating, but I promise it won't be as scary as you think. Even the people there wearing the most intense-looking spiked-leather underwear just want to have fun and play. Underneath the vinyl and leather, these might actually be your people. For more references to help find your kinky people, scan the QR code at the end of the book.

By now you may realize that you're at least a little bit kinkier than you thought. There is an exciting, diverse world of sex out there to be explored, and doing so can help you evolve your Sex IQ, heal some of your deepest wounds, and experience a whole lot of pleasure.

Now that your mind is open to sexual experiences that you may have never before considered, it's time to reach the final frontier...unconventional relationships.

10

New Ways to Relationship:

The Ins and Outs of Ethical Non-Monogamy

I have a confession to make. I was already late delivering this manuscript to my publisher (apologies again to my editor!) when I decided to add a chapter on ethical non-monogamy. Given the number of people who've been asking me about it lately, the book just felt incomplete without it.

More and more, people are coming to realize that love comes in many different ways, shapes, and forms. Historically, a "couple" meant a committed, monogamous relationship between two people of the opposite sex. Of course, many people still choose this arrangement, but for others it has become overly limiting. Gender norms have changed, and new and different types of non-monogamous relationships are quickly becoming more popular.

For many reasons, the assumption that monogamy is the norm is becoming outdated. Its history is rooted in patriarchal customs where women were the property of men, and monogamy made it easier to keep that property—and any offspring within a family unit. As we question some of these practices, unconventional relationships are slowly being accepted into the mainstream.

However, ethical non-monogamy is yet another aspect of sex that is widely misunderstood, even by people who consider themselves sex positive. It's absolutely true that non-monogamy isn't for everyone. But do you know what? Monogamy isn't for everyone, either!

Just look at the number of divorces and committed partners who cheat for evidence of this. It can be difficult to get accurate numbers on infidelity because studies rely on people to self-report, and not everyone wants to admit to an affair. Estimates of the number of people who cheat range from fifteen to forty-five percent of penis and vulva owners. Meanwhile, over twenty percent of people self-report that at some point they have been in an openly non-monogamous relationship.

If monogamy works for you, that's amazing. My goal here is not to try to convince you to explore non-monogamy if you don't want to. This is one area that should absolutely only be entered into by those who are completely, one hundred percent game. For this reason, a relationship with one partner that wants to ethically be non-monogamous and another who prefers monogamy is going to be extremely difficult for both parties.

My personal take is that monogamy and ethical non-monogamy are equally valid relationship models. The problem with monogamy isn't the model itself, but the fact that it's compulsory. When monogamy is a conscious choice, meaning that you've examined the other relationship models out there and done your internal work of understanding what you really need relationally and sexually to thrive, it can be fantastic. But if you've done all this work and come to the conclusion that it's not for you, ethical non-monogamy is also a valid choice. Of course, keep in mind that being married to more than one person is illegal. Outside of that, though, all forms of ethical (meaning all parties are aware, consenting, and informed) non-monogamy are fair game.

Consider this chapter a part of your relationship exploration. I'll help you understand these relationships better and hopefully destigmatize and demystify them for you. Of course, I'll also give you some advice around best practices for entering a healthy, happy ethically non-monogamous relationship if that's your choice. Maybe you'll decide to go for it, or maybe you'll just react more kindly when your niece tells you that she's in a triad or a throuple. Either way, it's a win!

At the end of the day, ethical non-monogamy still has a steep hill to climb when it comes to mainstream acceptance and recognition. But the more we can talk about alternate relationship models with nuance, respect, and curiosity, the more everyone benefits. Why? Because we can become more honest and open about love and sex in general and realize that we get to write our own life scripts, not just the ones that were handed to us by prior generations.

So, let's explore this new script together.

The Truth About Ethical Non-Monogamy

From the outset, I want to clear up any confusion about what non-monogamy is and what it is not. Ethical non-monogamy can include open relationships with one committed partner and then one or more sexual partners (like swinging), or more than one romantic and/or sexual partner, including husbands with boyfriends/girlfriends or wives with boyfriends/girlfriends. It's not simply a synonym for orgies or swinging.

While it often does include sex, this is not about orgasms or intercourse, per se. It's also not just for people who can't keep it in their pants, want an excuse to cheat, or aren't fully committed to their partners. In reality, most non-monogamous people have deep commitments to their partners, including a primary or anchor partner. They also tend to be extremely strong communicators and dedicate more time to talking and processing their feelings than they do having wild, nonstop sex. They generally spend more time talking and processing their feelings than most people in conventional relationships.

Does sex with multiple partners happen? Sometimes. Do orgasms happen? Hopefully! But for ethical non-monogamy to work peacefully, you really have to be on top of your communication game and be incredibly self-aware. In fact, many people find that they get to know themselves and their partners so much better through non-monogamy. Some even choose to pursue ethical non-monogamy specifically for this purpose.

Before getting involved in a non-monogamous relationship, be honest with yourself about your self-awareness, emotional regulation skills, and your ability to be open and vulnerable with your partner. Without these traits, non-monogamy may be difficult for you.

You also have to ask yourself honestly how important approval is to you. Many people in unconventional relationships struggle with the stigma. How will you feel if you face a backlash from your community for choosing this? What if your friends or family members openly disapprove? As a result of all this communication and self-reflection and getting to know each other, non-monogamous couples often find themselves getting closer after opening up their relationship instead of growing apart.

That said, non-monogamy is not a way to fix a relationship. If anything, it will put a spotlight on the problems in your current relationship, whether that's a lack of trust, a lack of connection, or an inability to communicate. This isn't always a bad thing, though. Once you are aware of these pain points, you can start to work on them—ideally before adding the complication of non-monogamy to the relationship.

Be honest with yourself and your partner about where you are in your relationship right now, particularly when it comes to trust. Without trust, non-monogamy will never work. Do you completely trust your partner to stick to the rules and boundaries you both agree to? This is key. Also ask yourself if there is a lot of conflict in your relationship. Do you feel emotionally safe with each other? Do you both want to do this for the same or similar reasons?

Another common myth is that non-monogamy is just for certain types of people—penis owners who have trouble being faithful, bisexuals, or those who are more spiritually evolved than the rest of us. We live in a patriarchal society, so it doesn't surprise me that some people assume that non-monogamy is just one more way for penis owners to win. But that's not what ethical non-monogamy is about.

My friend and fellow sex educator Wednesday Martin shared on my podcast that traditional monogamy is particularly rough on vulva owners' desire. Current primatology research reveals that many female primates strategically seek out multiple mates and probably have for eons. It sounds like vulva owners have evolved to desire sexual novelty. And today's vulva owners experience a huge drop in their desire for their partners within only one to four years in a relationship. Meanwhile, it takes penis owners nine to twelve years to experience the same drop. I was truly amazed to learn this!

This pattern has given rise to the harmful stereotype of the "frigid" wife. In heterosexual marriages, there is a false assumption that the wife is naturally less interested in sex than the husband. But research shows just the opposite. When they are allowed sexual variety in whatever form that might look like, married heterosexual women often become a lot more sexual in general. Let that sink in for a moment. All the tropes about men needing more sex than women are just plain wrong.

This simplified patriarchal view of non-monogamy extends to the myth that bisexual vulva owners are the only ones who seek it out. This falls under what I call the "necessary evil" justification for non-monogamy—in a heterosexual otherwise monogamous couple, the woman realizes she's bi, and her gracious male partner allows her to hook up with other women. How magnanimous!

The truth is, this is often a justification for what is known in non-monogamous circles as a "one penis policy." This is the idea that a woman can hook up outside of her heterosexual relationship, but only with fellow women. We rarely hear about a "one vulva policy" for penis owners, though, so we can very quickly see the imbalance here.

The fact is that people of all genders and sexual orientations choose non-monogamy. And it's not just for those who are "enlightened," either. In general, this lifestyle often attracts people who are comfortable challenging convention. But does that mean they're more enlightened, smarter, or "better" than monogamous people? Nope. Especially if those people have done the work of getting to know themselves and what they really want and need and decided to stick with monogamy from a conscious, intentional place.

So, what is ethical non-monogamy? It is a way of balancing variety and stability in our relationships. It is a way of expanding what it means to be a couple or to be in a committed relationship. And it is a way of continuing to make life adventurous and fun and to get our needs for intimacy, connection, and sexual expression met within the safe container of a supportive and mutually supportive relationship.

We can do this in many different ways.

Types of Non-Monogamy

While all non-monogamous relationships share certain things in common, there is no one-size-fits-all approach. Let's break down the different types of non-monogamous relationship styles.

Polyamory

Someone who is polyamorous is simultaneously in more than one romantic and/or sexual relationship at a time, always with the knowledge and consent of all partners. Everything is divulged, but the extent to which you share the details of your relationships with your other partners can vary. These relationships are not just limited to sex. They almost always include feelings of romance, love, and some level of commitment.

There are many different varieties of polyamorous relationships. You might have a primary or anchor partner plus one or more secondary or "side" partners that can also be romantic and/or more than just sexual. This is often called hierarchical polyamory because the primary or anchor partnership is prioritized above the others.

When I talked to Wednesday Martin about her experience with polyamory, she shared a story about her husband supporting her through a breakup with another partner. This might sound strange to some people, but I thought it was a beautiful example of love and commitment. Her husband is her primary partner. He is the priority. But she cared deeply about her other partner, and her husband was secure enough in their partnership to hold space for her very real feelings of loss.

There is also "nonhierarchical polyamory." In this case, there is no primary partnership. This can mean that you have more than one partner who are on equal footing. No one relationship is prioritized over another. This is similar to dating more than one person at a time, except everyone knows about each other, and those relationships tend to carry more of a commitment than a typical dating scenario.

Nonhierarchical polyamory can also mean there are more than two people in a serious relationship with each other at the same time. This is also known as a triad or "throuple" in the case of three partners, or a "quad" in the case of four partners. These are not conventional couples who invite a guest or guests to join them from time to time or even regularly. (Those couples might refer to themselves as swingers.) They are all equal members of the relationship. It's common for all members of a throuple or a quad to live together, though, again, it would be illegal for them to all be married.

Sometimes, the people in these relationships are open to adding another member if they meet the right person and all agree on it. Other times, the multiple partners are committed to each other and are not open to adding new partners. This is called polyfidelity. It is much like a closed monogamous relationship, just with more people.

Open Relationships

This is a catch-all term that covers a broad array of relationships. To be in an open relationship can mean many things. It can include polyamory, since those relationships are essentially open to others already. However, it can also mean that members of a primary partnership are free to seek sexual gratification with other partners. These side relationships may or may not include romantic feelings or any other aspects of a traditional relationship. An open relationship can also simply mean that a couple regularly invites one or more others to join them for a threesome or other form of group sex.

There are many ways to have an open relationship. It all depends on the people in the relationships and their needs and wants. Everyone involved must decide and discuss their boundaries, limitations, and needs.

Most people who opt for this arrangement might be considered emotionally mature. It's an expectation. It's not a part of the culture to treat people as disposable sex objects, even if they are just a guest who joins a couple for sex. This is about a mutual agreed-upon exchange of pleasure, whether the parties involved are looking for multiple partners, friends with benefits, or casual sex that's truly satisfying for everyone.

Apartnership

This is a relationship between two primary partners who are committed to each other but live apart, whether that's in separate spaces nearby or long-distance. Of course, this can be temporary or permanent.

Sometimes, people in apartnerships are in a monogamous relationship or even a marriage but live separately, either because of personal preference or other circumstances. This is also called Living Apart Together (LAT). There are people in apartnerships who agree to be polyamorous or to open the relationship while they are living apart, while others remain monogamous.

Swinging

Swinging can mean that two partners in a committed relationship exchange partners with another couple for a night to have sex, or it can involve large groups of couples getting together and swapping partners.

The main difference between swinging and being in an open relationship is that swingers usually share these erotic adventures. They may go off with different partners for the sex itself, but then they go home together. People in an open relationship, on the other hand, go off separately to have adventures that can include dates, trips, or just hookups with other people.

Swingers in particular have a robust community. There are clubs and cruises for swingers, and they often rent out restaurants or clubs for events. Sometimes, the couples who swing together develop friendships or swap with another couple multiple times, but the focus is always on the primary relationship.

Monogamish

Sex and relationship columnist Dan Savage coined the word "monogamish" to define a relationship that is like a traditional committed, monogamous relationship, except that the partners agree to step out sexually from time to time, such as when they are traveling or when they have group sex together.

The focus here is really on the primary relationship. Like in any type of open relationship, all of the other details really depend on the needs and boundaries of the people involved.

All of these types of relationships can merge and blend into one another. For example, a couple in an apartnership can also swing together when they're in the same location. People in a throuple or quad can also swing or open the relationship if they want to. And so on.

It's exciting to be able to write your own relationship rules, but it's essential that you and anyone that you are in a relationship with write those rules together so that it is safe and comfortable for everyone. To that end, let's discuss some things to think about first.

Before You Dive In

If you're curious about ethical non-monogamy and think you might want to give it a try, that's great. But I won't lie—this is tricky terrain that you shouldn't enter into lightly. It's important to go into this with your eyes wide-open and do some work beforehand to give yourself and your partner(s) the best possible chance of comfort, safety, and happiness.

Here are some of the steps you should take:

Know the Risks

The very idea of non-monogamy is triggering for many people. It touches on tender emotional territory, particularly for folks who have any type of fear of abandonment or have an anxious attachment style. Even if we grew up with stable caregivers and think of ourselves as open-minded, sexually liberated, confident people, we're marinated every day in the cultural belief that monogamy equals worthiness. The pinnacle of success is to get married, have a baby, and get that house! Therefore, we fear that if someone wants to be non-monogamous while in a relationship with us, it means that we're not enough—not hot enough, not interesting enough, not young enough, not great enough at sex, and on and on.

Non-monogamy can also trigger our deepest insecurities. What if you think your partner enjoys sex with someone else more than they do with you? What if you think their other partner is more attractive than you? What if they find more partners than you do?

Many people strike down the idea of non-monogamy because they can't imagine dealing with the feelings of jealousy. Just the thought of their partner being with someone else shuts the conversation down fast. Feeling jealous is painful. But here's the thing—we can and often do experience jealousy in both monogamous and non-monogamous relationships.

Jealousy can also be something to work on and lean into. It takes a lot of self-knowledge and self-acceptance to understand where our feelings of jealousy are coming from and do the inner work to change them. Jealousy can be a great teacher, and navigating this emotion can really help us understand ourselves and our partners better. When we're open and vulnerable about it with our partners, it can also enhance intimacy. Many people in non-monogamous relationships find that by doing this work over time, they are able to transform their feelings of jealousy into compersion, which is the ability to find joy in your partner's pleasure.

However, many people still don't think they could tolerate non-monogamy because of the fear that their primary partner will fall in love with someone else and maybe even leave them. The truth is, this is possible. But the deeper truth is, this is possible in any type of relationship, not just a non-monogamous one. People fall in love with others outside of their relationship and leave their partners all the time. Relationships are risky, period. The only difference here is that with non-monogamy, you're forced to face how risky they really are.

This can be deeply uncomfortable, but it can also force real growth and acceptance. It can also lead us to appreciate how precious our primary relationship is—we realize how badly we don't want to lose our primary partner. This can strengthen that relationship even more.

If you have kids, it's also important to think about how a non-monogamous relationship might affect them. I'm not saying that it's bad for kids, per se, to have caregivers in an unconventional relationship. It's good for kids to have happy, fulfilled caregivers. But it's important to consider how much about your relationships you are going to share with your kids and/or expose them to. Will they meet any partners outside of the primary relationship? Will any of your adventures take place in your home? How will you negotiate childcare among everyone involved?

Ultimately, children need stability, boundaries, and caregivers that love and care for them. If you make sure they have this, it is possible to maintain a healthy non-monogamous relationship without it affecting them negatively at all.

Try Other Forms of Novelty

Because non-monogamous relationships can be so tricky to navigate, it's worth taking the time to explore other ways of bringing a sense of novelty to your current relationship before giving it a try. Since some forms of non-monogamy can involve having novel sexual experiences, it is possible that adding something new will be enough to reinvigorate your sex life.

Ask yourself how you can mix things up in your sex life to bust out of your routine without bringing one or more new personalities into it. Think about everything you've learned so far in this book. Are there erogenous zones that are untapped? What about oral? Anal? A position you haven't tried? A kink that you want to explore? Buy a massage candle or play with new toys. Read erotica to each other about having threesomes. Watch threesome porn.

I once spoke to a couple that felt that their sex life had grown stale and were seriously considering having a threesome. I encouraged them to first try watching threesome porn together and role-playing a threesome. They were shocked by how hot it was, and as it became a part of their sexual repertoire, they realized that it was a fantasy they didn't need to experience in real life.

If you've tried adding novelty to your sex life and are certain that you want to proceed, the next step can be a tricky one.

Talk to Your Partner

Asking your partner to open up your relationship in any way might feel like the most loaded request you can make. It can trigger all of their deepest insecurities and fears of abandonment. They might think that you don't want to be with them anymore, aren't attracted to them anymore, or that this is just a half step toward leaving the relationship for someone else. Or, they might surprise you and be excited and feel on the same page. Regardless, you want to tread very lightly.

It's especially important here to follow all of the communication rules. Wait until you're out of the bedroom to bring it up. When you're both feeling relaxed and close, you can try starting small. Say something like, "I feel so secure and happy in our relationship that I'm comfortable talking to you about something I've been fantasizing about. We've watched threesome porn, and I think it would be so hot to give it a try. It's something I'm interested in exploring together, but only if you're into it."

Or say something about why you think it would be hot for you as a couple: "I know you've been turned on by watching other women. I think it would be so hot to see you with someone else giving you pleasure."

This makes it clear that your partner is your priority. You're not cheating, and you're not unsatisfied. Instead, you're interested in pursuing this together.

See how they react, but if they don't respond or say no, drop it. Wait a little while for the other person to raise the topic again. I promise they didn't forget. If they don't bring it up, it's because they don't want to pursue it. In this case, silence is your answer. Don't push it with consent or boundaries. This may lead to a big fight or a deep wound.

After some time passes, though, you can try bringing it up again. Remember, this isn't something you want to rush into, so use that time to try to bring novelty into your sex life in other ways and/or to research non-monogamous relationships and make sure they're right for you.

If, after all that, you still want to move forward, you can try to bring it up again. Say something like, "I know I've mentioned it before, and I don't want to push you, but I've been thinking more about the threesome idea and even did some research. If you're open to it, there are all kinds of other things we could try." (Of course, you can replace "threesome" here with "open relationship," "polyamory," etc.)

Share what you've learned, paying attention to your partner's verbal and physical cues. If they shut down or are nonreceptive, it's time to let this go. Non-monogamy is not for everyone, and if your partner is not interested, you have to respect that. In order for this to work, both partners need to be one hundred percent on board.

If you do get some interest and your partner comes back to you with a yes or a maybe, the conversation can continue slowly, with empathy and openness. Remember when I said that there was a lot of talking involved in non-monogamy? It's just as important to continue using your best communication skills after you get a yes to discuss how this is going to potentially work.

Set Rules

Ironically, opening up a relationship can mean setting more rules and boundaries than keeping it monogamous. Every facet of non-monogamy needs to be unpacked slowly and agreed upon. How will it go down? (Will you?) What is "allowed," and what's off-limits?

The most important thing here is to never assume what your partner wants or is okay with. Always ask. You might think it's obvious that you or your partner would never sleep with someone within your social circle, while they might be thrilled to finally be able to have sex with their hot friend. Or you might assume that you'll fill each other in on all the details of your adventures because you get turned on by hearing about your partner being with someone else, while they'd prefer a policy of "Don't ask, don't tell."

Any of these misassumptions can lead to the breakdown of a relationship. Don't let that happen. You can avoid this by setting extremely clear rules and boundaries and thoroughly discussing them. It's just as important to understand why your partner does or doesn't want to agree to a rule as it is to set the rule. Like I said, a lot of talking.

This process might also involve some level of negotiation. Your partner might want to set a rule that you can only see someone once, while you may want it to be five times. Hopefully, you can compromise and set a rule that it's three times and they're out. Just remember that you're on the same team here. You're not negotiating with an opponent. If it ever feels that way, you might want to step back and reconsider. The goal is to find ways to make sure you both get what you want and need while preserving the relationship.

Even if you're having a simple threesome or swinging together, rules are still important. First of all, who are you going to do this with? Will it be someone you already know? Will they spend the night? Will you keep in touch after? Will there be snack breaks?

Here are some examples of rules that you might want to set. Use this list as inspiration, but also think deeply about what might come up later and add some rules of your own. The more you can anticipate issues and set rules around them before they rear their ugly heads, the better off you'll be.

- Are you allowed to kiss other people?

- Exactly which sex acts are okay and which aren't?

- Can you go out on dates with other people, or just have sex?

- Will you always use condoms or another form of protection when having penetrative sex with another person?

- Are you allowed to continue seeing someone that you've developed feelings for?
- Will you see people that either of you already knows (someone in your social circle or who you work with)?
- Can you bring people back to your home? What about your bed?
- Will you check in with each other while you're out with someone else? How often?
- Are you going to spend the night with other people?
- How many times will you see someone?
- Will you share details of your adventures with each other? What kind of details?
- Do the same rules apply when you're traveling?
- Will you see penis owners, vulva owners, or both?

Revisit Those Rules

Yep, it's time for more talking. The most successful couples set rules before heading out on their adventures and then revisit and adapt these rules as time goes on. Your needs and your partner's will change over time, and so will the things you're comfortable with. The ground is always moving beneath your feet, and you have to keep an open mind for things to change. This is true in any relationship, but in non-monogamous relationships it tends to move faster.

Decide beforehand when you'll revisit the rules—in a week, a month, six months, a year? Then sit down together when the time comes, and be honest with each other about what worked for you and what didn't. Are there rules you want to change or add? Or do you want to close the relationship again and go back to monogamy, either temporarily or permanently?

I once spoke to a couple who wanted to open their relationship. They talked it through, they set the rules, and they started off with a really fun and hot threesome. When they talked about it after, they both felt like that one experience was enough to reignite their sex life. They stayed monogamous and shared joint fantasies about it for years.

For this couple, breaking down the barrier just once was enough. It deepened their connection, and they had an awesome time. Rather than take another risk of potential jealousy and pressure, they decided to quit while they were ahead.

Of course, I know plenty of other couples who have gone the other way. They started off with what they thought would be a onetime thing but ended up liking it so much that they decided to add someone to their relationship and become a closed throuple. Others agreed to open up the relationship completely and both start seeing other people. It's also common for couples to close and reopen their relationship periodically, based on how they are feeling about things at the time. Change is inevitable, and when you write your own relationships rules it can be very exciting!

Whether or not you ever consider opening your relationship or pursuing non-monogamy, it's great to know all of the options instead of just assuming that traditional monogamy is the only way. That's kind of like assuming that "conventional sex" is the only way to seek pleasure!

By now, I hope you know that there is a long, diverse menu of options out there when it comes to pleasure, sex, and relationships. You get to choose from that menu for yourself. You can even start from scratch and create your own menu. Then, I encourage you to order up. Take a nibble of one appetizer, and if you don't like it, try something else next.

As you taste and explore new things, you'll grow your Sex IQ, and as you grow your Sex IQ, you'll learn more and more about what brings you the greatest possible amounts of happiness, fulfilment, and pleasure. Which is exactly what you deserve.

CONCLUSION

Own Your Pleasure

After almost twenty years of hosting my podcast, *Sex With Emily*, it's fascinating to see that the questions people ask me the most frequently haven't changed. Not one bit. Every single day, there's a vulva owner who has never had an orgasm, a partner in a long-term relationship who wants to spice it up, or a penis owner who's deeply ashamed of their performance in the bedroom. And while I love nothing more than arming people with the knowledge they seek to make their lives more pleasurable, my greatest hope is that by reading this book you will learn to evolve and regulate and understand your Sex IQ enough to start answering these questions—and more—for yourself.

The next time you're not in the mood for sex (and it will happen!) you can run through the pillars of Sex IQ and come up with your own answers for why you might not be feeling turned-on that day. Talk about sexual liberation! This is how we will evolve the conversation around sex and go even deeper.

My goal for you is to use your Sex IQ to not just become a better lover, but also to reframe the way you think about sex and intimate relationships and what it means to be a good lover to begin with. Giving and receiving pleasure and being "good in bed" have nothing to do with your age, your body type, your penis size, your sexual history, or your number of orgasms. It's about being smart about sex.

As you evolve your Sex IQ, you will discover a new way of being in the world. I also hope that you will begin to use it as a tool to evaluate and understand yourself and even your partners and potential partners from a place of acceptance and love. If I could go back in time with a greater Sex IQ, I would make very different decisions. I would have more difficult conversations, ask for what I really want in bed, and make room for a lot more pleasure. Remember that you're responsible for your own pleasure and knowing what feels good, so make decisions based on how you feel. I hope that you will allow this to guide you moving forward. It has the potential to change your entire life.

In the academic and scientific worlds, sex has never been recognized as an integral or even related part of overall health, but it's finally beginning to gain more acceptance. We know that your sexual health impacts every area of your life, and that every other area of your life affects how you show up in your intimate relationships. Therefore, the knowledge in this book has unlimited potential to holistically improve your life and well-being.

I'm excited for you to be on this journey, no matter where you're starting from. Developing your sexual intelligence takes time, commitment, and consistency. Be patient with yourself. And enjoy using this new arsenal of skills to build your relationships, your confidence, your connection to your body, and your pleasure.

Sex is an ever-evolving and emerging field of study, and your personal work is ongoing, too. I hope you'll continue to use this book as a resource and stay connected. I will provide you with the most up-to-date information to evolve your Sex IQ on my website.

Most of all, I want you to know that your pleasure is not something that you have to sit back and wait for or rely on anyone else to give to you. You are in control of your own sexual destiny. Pleasure is productivity. Pleasure is presence, and pleasure is your birthright. I'm so excited for you to claim all that is rightfully yours.

★★★★★

RESOURCES

Education Sources

- AfroSexology: https://afrosexology.com/
- EDSE (Everyone Deserves Sex Ed.): https://everyonedeservessexed.com/
- The Gottman Institute: https://www.gottman.com/
- Scarleteen: https://www.scarleteen.com/
- Sex Positive Families: https://sexpositivefamilies.com/
- Sex With Emily: www.sexwithemily.com
- Somatica: https://www.somaticainstitute.com/somatica-philosophy/
- OMGYes: https://start.omgyes.com/

Books

These are my top recommendation for doctors and writers on sexual health and wellness:

- *Better Sex Through Mindfulness: How Women Can Cultivate Desire* by Lori A. Brotto, PhD
- *Pleasure Activism* by Adrienne Maree Brown
- *Urban Tantra* by Barbara Carrellas
- *Curvy Girl Sex* by Elle Chase
- *Sex, When You Don't Feel Like It: The Truth About Mismatched Libido & Rediscovering Desire* by Cyndi Darnell
- *Sex for One* by Betty Dodson
- *Prostate Health* by Charlie Glickman
- *She Comes First: The Thinking Man's Guide to Pleasuring a Woman* by Ian Kerner, PhD
- *How To Do the Work, Recognize Your Patterns, Heal from Your Past and Create Yourself* by Dr. Nicole LePera
- *Untrue: Why Nearly Everything We Believe About Women, Lust, and Infidelity is Wrong and How the New Science Can Set Us Free* by Wednesday Martin
- *Cliterate* by Dr. Laurie Mintz
- *Come as You Are: The Surprising New Science that Will Transform Your Sex Life* by Emily Nagoski, PhD
- *Mating in Captivity* by Esther Perel

- *What Makes a Baby* by Cory Silverberg
- *Read Me: A Parental Primer for "The Talk"* by Lanae St. John
- *The Ultimate Guide to Anal Sex for Women* by Tristan Taormino
- *Unbound: A Woman's Guide to Power* by Kasia Urbaniak
- *The Body Keeps the Score* by Bessel A. Van der Kolk
- *Women's Anatomy of Arousal* by Sheri Winston

These are my top recommendations for doctors and writers on hormone health:

- *Your Body in Balance* by Dr. Neal Barnard
- *Beyond the Pill: A 30-Day Program to Balance Your Hormones, Reclaim Your Body, and Reverse the Dangerous Side Effects of the Birth Control Pill* by Dr. Jolene Brighten
- *The Menopause Manifesto: Own Your Health with Facts and Feminism* by Dr. Jen Gunter
- *Menopause Bootcamp* by Suzanne Gilberg-Lenz, MD
- *Testosterone for Life: Recharge Your Sex Drive, Muscle Mass, Energy and Overall Health* by Abraham Morgentaler
- *Hormone Intelligence: The Complete Guide to Calming Hormone Chaos and Restoring Your Body's Natural Blueprint for Well-Being* by Aviva Romm, MD

Ethical porn and erotica websites and apps:

- Bellesa: https://www.bellesa.co/

- Dipsea: https://www.dipseastories.com/
- Erika Lust: https://erikalust.com/
- Lady Cheeky: https://ladycheeky.newtumbl.com/
- MakeLoveNotPorn: https://makelovenotporn.tv/
- Pink & White Productions: https://pinkwhite.biz/
- Quinn: https://www.tryquinn.com/

Visit my website, sexwithemily.com, and listen to my podcast, *Sex with Emily*, for loads of additional information, including a list of sex educators and therapists and recommendations about pleasure products and sex accessories. We continue to update this list regularly.

REFERENCES

Roberts S. C., Klapilová K., Little A. C., Burriss R. P., Jones B. C., DeBruine L. M, Petrie M., Havlícek J. "Relationship satisfaction and outcome in women who meet their partner while using oral contraception." *Proc Biol Sci.* 2012 Apr 7; 279(1732):1430-6. doi: 10.1098/rspb.2011.1647. Epub 2011 Oct 12. PMID: 21993500; PMCID: PMC3282363.

Adlercreutz H., Pulkkinen M. O., Hämäläinen E. K., and Korpela J. T. (1984). "Studies on the role of intestinal bacteria in metabolism of synthetic and natural steroid hormones." J. Steroid Biochem. 20, 217–229. doi: 10.1016/0022-4731(84)90208-5.

Flores R., Shi J., Fuhrman B., Xu X., Veenstra T. D., Gail, M. H., et al. (2012). "Fecal microbial determinants of fecal and systemic estrogens and estrogen metabolites: a cross-sectional study." J. Transl. Med. 10:253. doi: 10.1186/1479-5876-10-253.

Khalili H. "Risk of Inflammatory Bowel Disease with Oral Contraceptives and Menopausal Hormone Therapy: Current

Evidence and Future Directions." *Drug Saf.* 2016 Mar;39(3):193-7. doi: 10.1007/s40264-015-0372-y. PMID: 26658991; PMCID: PMC4752384.

Shackleton C. H. "Role of a disordered steroid metabolome in the elucidation of sterol and steroid biosynthesis." *Lipids.* 2012;47(1):1-12. doi:10.1007/s11745-011-3605-6.

Bekhbat M., Neigh G. N. "Sex differences in the neuro-immune consequences of stress: Focus on depression and anxiety." *Brain Behav Immun.* 2018 Jan; 67:1-12. doi: 10.1016/j.bbi.2017.02.006. Epub 2017 Feb 16. PMID: 28216088; PMCID: PMC5559342.

Brody S., Krüger T. H. "The post-orgasmic prolactin increase following intercourse is greater than following masturbation and suggests greater satiety." *Biol Psychol.* 2006 Mar;71(3):312-5. doi: 10.1016/j.biopsycho.2005.06.008. Epub 2005 Aug 10. PMID: 16095799.

Hoz, F. J. (2017). "PM-05 Prevalence and Characterization of Female Ejaculation. Cross-sectional Study." *The Journal of Sexual Medicine.* 14. e382. 10.1016/j.jsxm.2017.10.044.

Wimpissinger F., Springer C., Stackl W. "International online survey: female ejaculation has a positive impact on women's and their partners' sexual lives." *BJU Int.* 2013 Jul;112(2):E177-85. doi: 10.1111/j.1464-410X.2012.11562.x. Epub 2013 Jan 25. PMID: 23350685.

Liu H., Shen S., Hsieh N. "A National Dyadic Study of Oral Sex, Relationship Quality, and Well-Being among Older Couples." J Gerontol B Psychol Sci Soc Sci. 2019;74(2):298-308. doi:10.1093/geronb/gby089

Moran C., Lee C. "What's normal? Influencing women's perceptions of normal genitalia: an experiment involving exposure to modified and nonmodified images." *BJOG*. 2014 May;121(6):761-6. doi: 10.1111/1471-0528.12578. Epub 2013 Dec 19. PMID: 24354731.

Scan this QR code for up-to-date resources and references to boost your Sex IQ.

ACKNOWLEDGMENTS

When I embarked on this career almost twenty years ago, it wasn't cool or socially acceptable to talk about sex unless it was Dr. Ruth Westheimer, so thank you to the pioneer for paving the way and allowing me to see this path was possible.

It's one thing to be talking about sex all these years—it's a whole other thing to write it all down. Thank you to my writing partner, Jodi Lipper—I couldn't have created this book without you. Thank you for your extraordinary expertise.

To my editor, Erika Imranyi—thank you for your meticulous and wise counsel, and for believing in me and this book. Thank you to the whole team at Park Row Books and HarperCollins.

Thank you to my agent, Brandi Bowles, for your knowledge and guidance during this process and thank you to my entire team at United Talent Agency. Thank you also to my fabulous illustrator, Priscilla Witte, for your detailed and memorable illustrations.

Thank you to my friend Anne Hodder-Shipp for your careful review and help with the manuscript. Thank you, Tolly Mosely, for your creativity, passion, and loving contribution early on, and to Val Frankel for your help, as well.

I want to thank my colleagues, mentors, and friends in the sexual health, education, and pleasure space. Together we are daring to break new ground.

Thank you to Esther Perel for making the topic of intimacy more intelligent and engaging.

I've learned and experienced so much alongside Celeste Hirschman and Danielle Harrell, Pamela Madsen, Dolly Josette and John Wineland, Jamye Waxman, and Dr. Hernando Chaves. Thank you for being generous with your knowledge.

Thank you to the *Sex with Emily* team for your support, dedication, and hard work in getting my message out into the world. It truly takes a village.

Thanks to my radio family and friends, Dr. Drew Pinsky, and Menace. Some of my most favorite career highlights are with you.

Thank you to Mary P., Lisa Levens, and Lisa Campbell, for your unwavering support, love, and keeping all my secrets the last thirty years (that will be the next book). Our decades-long friendship is one of my greatest joys and achievements. Thank you, Charlotte Rubin, for your loyal presence. You make my life way more entertaining.

Thank you, Elle Chase—I love you more than you love David Bowie. Thank you to my soul sister Jennifer Freed, for being a steady presence and source of wisdom and thoughtful guidance. Thank you to my friend Wednesday Martin for your thoughtfulness and inspiring me to leave the house during the writing process.

Thank you, Sarah Brokaw, for always being a source of stability and fun, a winning combination. Thank you, Jennifer Cohen, president of my "bold" of directors; Adrienne Arieff for your love, support, and feeling like home; Chelsey Goodan, thank you for being so supportive, reading the early version of the manuscript.

Thank you to Matthew for being so loving, supportive, and sexy during the book process and in my life, because "research is me-search."

To my furry little Jojo for reminding me that life is about finding pleasure every day—long walks, belly rubs, and staying under the covers as long as possible.

Finally, thanks to my family, my mom, and my bonus dad, Ed, for being so loving, supportive, and always a good time. To my nieces Jillian, Ella, and Lexie—you're the reason I want a positive sex culture. Thank you for inspiring me every day. I love you.